# Rabbit Medicine and Surgery for Veterinary Nurses

# Rabbit Medicine and Surgery for Veterinary Nurses

**Mary A. Fraser**

BVMS, PhD, CertVD, PGCHE, FHEA, CBiol, MIBiol, MRCVS

*Lecturer, Veterinary Nursing, Napier University, Edinburgh*

**Simon J. Girling**

BVMS(Hons), DZooMed, CBiol, MIBiol, MRCVS

*RCVS Specialist in Zoo Animal and Wildlife Medicine*

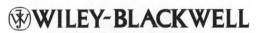

A John Wiley & Sons, Ltd., Publication

This edition first published 2009
© 2009 by Mary A. Fraser and Simon J. Girling

Blackwell Publishing was acquired by John Wiley & Sons in February 2007.
Blackwell's publishing programme has been merged with Wiley's global Scientific,
Technical, and Medical business to form Wiley-Blackwell.

*Registered office*
John Wiley & Sons Ltd, The Atrium, Southern Gate, Chichester, West Sussex, PO19 8SQ,
United Kingdom

*Editorial offices*
9600 Garsington Road, Oxford, OX4 2DQ, United Kingdom
2121 State Avenue, Ames, Iowa 50014-8300, USA

For details of our global editorial offices, for customer services and for information about
how to apply for permission to reuse the copyright material in this book please see our
website at www.wiley.com/wiley-blackwell.

The right of the author to be identified as the author of this work has been asserted in
accordance with the Copyright, Designs and Patents Act 1988.

*Library of Congress Cataloging-in-Publication Data*
Fraser, Mary A.
  Rabbit medicine and surgery for veterinary nurses / Mary A. Fraser, Simon J. Girling.
     p. ; cm.
  Includes bibliographical references and index.
  ISBN 978-1-4051-4706-4 (pbk. : alk. paper)    1. Rabbits–Diseases. 2. Rabbits–Surgery. 3.
Rabbits–Health. 4. Rabbits.    I. Girling, Simon. II. Title.
  [DNLM:   1. Animal Diseases–nursing. 2. Rabbits. 3. Animal Husbandry–methods.
4. Animal Technicians. 5. Surgical Procedures, Operative–veterinary. 6. Veterinary
Medicine–methods.    SF 997.5.R2 F842r 2009]
  SF997.5.R2F73 2009
  636.932'2–dc22                                                        2008028176

A catalogue record for this book is available from the British Library.

Set in 10/13pt Palatino by Aptara® Inc., New Delhi, India

1   2009

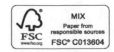

# Contents

*Colour plates appear between pages 104 and 105*

v

# Foreword

Rabbits are now the third most common pet in the UK – and becoming ever more popular. Over the years rabbits have moved from pets kept in the back garden through to animals that now often live in the house alongside other pets and their owners.

The role of the veterinary nurse in practice has also changed in recent years, with nurses now having a much more defined role and having more responsibility for their patients and the care they give. The use of nursing care plans is only one example of how veterinary nursing has its own specifically defined role in veterinary practice rather than just following on from the work of the veterinary surgeon.

The aim of this book is to provide veterinary nurses with an easy to read source of information about rabbits. Everyone reading this book will come with a different level of knowledge about rabbits but we hope that there will be something useful for everyone.

Mary A. Fraser
Simon J. Girling

# Rabbits – A Natural History

## 1.1 The wild rabbit and natural behaviour

### 1.1.1 The wild rabbit

The wild rabbit (*Oryctolagus cuniculus*) was thought to have been introduced to mainland UK by the Normans. However, there is some evidence that the Romans may have brought them over from the continent a thousand years earlier. Originally, *O. cuniculus* was kept and bred for meat and fur, often being kept over large areas of land, and may have been first domesticated in Italy or North Africa from Roman times or even earlier. The Romans used to keep rabbits in large walled areas of ground that allowed the rabbit to form natural warren systems – a feature copied in Britain in the Middle Ages. The wild form of *O. cuniculus* has been discovered in fossilised forms in Western Europe, chiefly in Spain and Southern France. Indeed, the name 'Spain' may have originally derived from the Phoenician name for that area, which literally translated means 'land of the rabbits' (Okerman, 1994). Since its introduction to mainland Britain *O. cuniculus* has been bred prior to the eighteenth century chiefly for meat, with its pelt being used as a by-product for clothing. Even after the time when the fashion for breeding rabbits for their appearance emerged, the domestic rabbit has still been kept as a prolific source of food in the UK, as witnessed by the wide-scale keeping of rabbits by British families during the two world wars of the twentieth century, for example. The breeding of fancy rabbits in the eighteenth century though resulted in the development of many of the breeds that are kept and showed as pet rabbits today.

## 1.1.2 Taxonomy

Rabbits belong to the order Lagomorpha. The order Lagomorpha is separated from the order Rodentia by a number of features: the most obvious being the extra pair of maxillary incisors, which in lagomorphs are positioned immediately behind the main maxillary incisors (the so-called peg teeth). However, the separation between the two orders (once lagomorphs were thought to be a subdivision of Rodentia) is deeper than this, and serological studies (Moody *et al.*, 1949) have shown no closer affinity between lagomorphs and rodents than between many other mammalian orders.

The order Lagomorpha comprises two families: Leporidae and Ochotonidae. The family Leporidae includes the genus *Lepus* to which hares belong (e.g. *Lepus europaeus*, the brown hare and *Lepus timidus*, the Arctic hare) and the genus *Oryctolagus* to which European rabbits belong (*O. cuniculus*). The family Leporidae also contains the genus *Sylvilagus* to which the cottontail rabbits of the New World belong. Cottontails are generally more solitary than *O. cuniculus* and do not create burrows. The family Ochotonidae contains the Afghan (*Ochotona rufescens*) and Colorado/American (*Ochotona princeps*) pikas amongst others. These are also known as conies or mouse hares due to their more rodent-like body form and short ears. Further classification of the order Lagomorpha is given in Table 1.1.

As you can see from Table 1.1, rabbits found in North and South America are related to the British rabbit, but there are a number of different species of American rabbits. Within the genus *Sylvilagus* there is a great deal of diversity in the appearance of these rabbits. Some such as the desert cottontail (*Sylvilagus audubonii*) resemble the European brown hare (*L. europaeus*) in their larger appearance, longer legs, and in their tendency to live above ground rather than in a burrow, although they are still classified as a rabbit rather than a hare. In comparison to this the eastern cottontail (*Sylvilagus floridanus*) looks similar to *O. cuniculus*.

The pikas bear very little physical similarities to the rabbit. Indeed, they look more like large hamsters than rabbits, being 12–25 cm in length with short, rounded ears. They also have other unusual anatomical differences in that the males do not possess a scrotum and the females do not possess a vulva, instead a cloaca-like structure exists in both sexes. In addition, their dental formula is different from rabbits and hares. Rabbits and hares have a dental formula of I 2/1, C 0/0, Pm 3/2, M 3/3, whereas the pikas have a formula of I 2/1, C 0/0, Pm 3/2, M 2/3 (where I, incisors; C, canines; Pm, premolars; and M, molars).

**Table 1.1** Classification of some of the order Lagomorpha with reference to the families Leporidae and Ochotonidae

| Phylum | Class | Order | Family | Genus | Species | English name |
|---|---|---|---|---|---|---|
| Chordata | Mammalia | Lagomorpha | Leporidae | Lepus | alleni | Antelope jackrabbit (USA and Mexico) |
| | | | | Lepus | americanus | Snowshoe hare (North America) |
| | | | | Lepus | arcticus | Canadian arctic hare (Canada and Greenland) |
| | | | | Lepus | brachyurus | Japanese hare (Japan) |
| | | | | Lepus | californicus | Black-tailed jackrabbit (USA) |
| | | | | Lepus | callotis | White-sided jackrabbit (USA and Mexico) |
| | | | | Lepus | capensis | Cape hare (South Africa) |
| | | | | Lepus | castroviejoi | Broom hare (Spain) |
| | | | | Lepus | commus | Yunna hare (China) |
| | | | | Lepus | coreanus | Korean hare (China and Korea) |
| | | | | Lepus | corsicanus | Corsican hare (Italy and Corsica) |
| | | | | Lepus | europaeus | Brown hare (Europe) |
| | | | | Lepus | fagani | Ethiopian hare (Ethiopia and Somalia) |
| | | | | Lepus | flavigularis | Tehuantepec hare/jackrabbit (Mexico) |
| | | | | Lepus | granatensis | Granada hare (Spain and Portugal) |
| | | | | Lepus | hainanas | Hainan hare (China) |
| | | | | Lepus | insularis | Black jackrabbit (Mexico) |
| | | | | Lepus | mandscharicus | Manchurian hare (China and Russia) |
| | | | | Lepus | nigricollis | Indian hare (India, Pakistan and Indonesia) |
| | | | | Lepus | oiostolus | Woolly hare (India and China) |
| | | | | Lepus | othus | Alaskan hare (USA and Russia) |
| | | | | Lepus | peguensis | Burmese hare (Cambodia, Thailand and Vietnam) |
| | | | | Lepus | saxatilis | Scrub hare (South Africa) |
| | | | | Lepus | sinensis | Chinese hare (China, Vietnam and Taiwan) |
| | | | | Lepus | starcki | Ethiopian highland hare (Ethiopia) |
| | | | | Lepus | timidus | Arctic hare (North Europe and Russia) |
| | | | | Lepus | tolai | Tolai hare (Russia, India, China, Afghanistan and Iran) |
| | | | | Lepus | townsendii | White-tailed jackrabbit (USA) |
| | | | | Lepus | victoriae | Savannah hare (West, Central and South Africa) |

(continued)

**Table 1.1** (Continued)

| Phylum | Class | Order | Family | Genus | Species | English name |
|---|---|---|---|---|---|---|
| | | | | *Lepus* | *yarkandensis* | Yarkland hare (China) |
| | | | | *Oryctolagus* | *cuniculus* | European rabbit |
| | | | | *Nesolagus* | *netscheri* | Sumatran rabbit (Indonesia) |
| | | | | *Nesolagus* | *timminsi* | Annamite striped rabbit (Vietnam) |
| | | | | *Pentalagus* | *furnessi* | Amami rabbit (Japan) |
| | | | | *Poelagus* | *marjorita* | Central African grass rabbit (Central Africa) |
| | | | | *Pronolagus* | *crassicaudatus* | Natal red hare (South Africa) |
| | | | | *Pronolagus* | *randensis* | Jameson's red rock hare (South Africa) |
| | | | | *Pronolagus* | *rupestris* | Common red rock rabbit (South Africa) |
| | | | | *Romerolagus* | *diazi* | Volcano rabbit (Mexico) |
| | | | | *Sylvilagus* | *aquaticus* | Swamp rabbit (USA) |
| | | | | *Sylvilagus* | *audubonii* | Desert cottontail (USA and Mexico) |
| | | | | *Sylvilagus* | *bachmani* | Brush rabbit (USA) |
| | | | | *Sylvilagus* | *brasiliensis* | Tapeti (Central and South America) |
| | | | | *Sylvilagus* | *cognatus* | Manzano Mountain cottontail (USA) |
| | | | | *Sylvilagus* | *cunicularis* | Mexican cottontail (Mexico) |
| | | | | *Sylvilagus* | *dicei* | Dice's cottontail (Central America) |
| | | | | *Sylvilagus* | *floridanus* | Eastern cottontail (USA) |
| | | | | *Sylvilagus* | *graysoni* | Tres Maria cottontail (Mexico) |
| | | | | *Sylvilagus* | *nuttallii* | Mountain cottontail (North America) |
| | | | | *Sylvilagus* | *mansuetus* | San José brush rabbit (Mexico) |
| | | | | *Sylvilagus* | *obscurus* | Appalachian cottontail (USA) |
| | | | | *Sylvilagus* | *palustris* | Marsh rabbit (USA) |
| | | | | *Sylvilagus* | *transitionalis* | New England cottontail (USA) |
| | | | | *Sylvilagus* | *varynaensis* | Barinas rabbit (Venezuela) |
| | | | Ochotonidae | *Ochotona* | *alpina* | Alpine pika (Russia, China and Mongolia) |
| | | | | *Ochotona* | *argentata* | Silver pika (China) |
| | | | | *Ochotona* | *cansus* | Gansa pika (China) |

| | | |
|---|---|---|
| Ochotona | collaris | Alaskan pika (North America) |
| Ochotona | curzoniae | Black-lipped pika (Russia, Mongolia and China) |
| Ochotona | daurica | Daurian pika (Russia, Mongolia and China) |
| Ochotona | erythrotis | Chinese red pika (China) |
| Ochotona | forresti | Forrest's pika (India, China and Bhutan) |
| Ochotona | gaoligongensis | Gaoligong pika (China) |
| Ochotona | gloveri | Glover's pika (China) |
| Ochotona | himalayana | Himalayan pika (Tibet and China) |
| Ochotona | hoffmanni | Hoffmann's pika (Russia and Mongolia) |
| Ochotona | huangensis | Tsing-Ling pika (China) |
| Ochotona | hyperborea | Northern pika (Russia, Mongolia and China) |
| Ochotona | iliensis | Ilia pika (China) |
| Ochotona | koslowi | Kozolv's pika (China) |
| Ochotona | ladacensis | Ladakh pika (India, Pakistan and China) |
| Ochotona | lama | Lama pika (Nepal) |
| Ochotona | macrotis | Large-eared pika (China, India, Pakistan and Afghanistan) |
| Ochotona | muliensis | Muli pika (China) |
| Ochotona | nigritia | Piamma black pika (China) |
| Ochotona | pallasi | Pallas's pika (Russia, Mongolia, China and Kazakhstan) |
| Ochotona | princeps | American pika coney or rock rabbit (USA) |
| Ochotona | pusilla | Steppe pika (Russia) |
| Ochotona | roylei | Royle's pika (China, India and Pakistan) |
| Ochotona | rufescens | Afghan pika |
| Ochotona | rutila | Turkestan red pika (Afghanistan, Kazakhstan, Tazikistan and Uzbekistan) |
| Ochotona | thibetana | Moupin pika (India and China) |
| Ochotona | thomasi | Thomas's pika (China) |
| Ochotona | turuchanensis | Turuchan pika (Russia) |

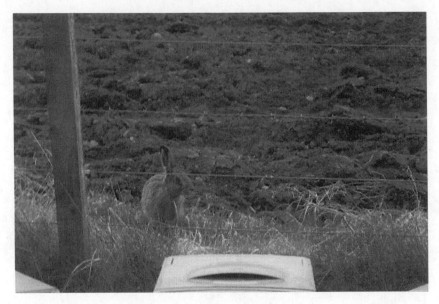

**Figure 1.1** Photograph of a hare.

Pikas also have a very high normal average body temperature of 40.1°C (104.2°F).

## 1.1.3 Rabbits and hares

Many characteristics are shared between rabbits and hares, such as their general appearance (see Fig. 1.1), dentition and eating habits, but there are also some significant differences. The main differences are listed in Table 1.2.

**Table 1.2** Comparison of physical features of rabbits and hares

| Feature | Rabbit | Hare |
| --- | --- | --- |
| Size | Smaller | Larger |
| Length of legs | Short hindlimbs | Longer hindlimbs |
| Ears | Short ears, usually held close to body | Long ears, with black tips, usually erect |
| Burrowing | *Oryctolagus* spp. burrow avidly. Some *Sylvilagus* spp. do not burrow | *Lepus* spp. do not burrow |
| Running stamina | Generally poor over distances | Adapted for longer distance flight and one of the fastest land animals in the UK |

The rest of this chapter deals only with the species *O. cuniculus* except where specifically stated.

### 1.1.4 Natural behaviour of rabbits

Rabbits are gregarious animals preferring to live in the company of others. In the wild they loosely live in large warrens that can contain up to 60–70 individuals. Within this warren, rabbits will live in closer smaller groups – either in a male/female pair or more commonly in groups of between 2 and 8 individuals. Within these groups a hierarchy exists where male animals will not tolerate the presence of other males and so older males will drive out younger ones. Generally, a dominant male rabbit (or 'buck') will choose a female rabbit (or 'doe') as a permanent mate. The more dominant males will also mate with one or more additional does as a sort of harem. The tunnels are dug by the pregnant does to provide nests for parturition.

Rabbits create a specific toilet area for faeces and urine and so are relatively easy to house/litter train. However, entire bucks will territory mark with urine and scent gland secretions (see below).

In the wild, rabbits can live until 8 years old, although predation and road casualties often results in the death of rabbits at a much younger age than this.

Although pet rabbits are somewhat removed from wild rabbits in their appearance, the behaviour of the wild rabbits and that of the pet can often be very similar. Many of the conditions that are encountered in pet rabbits can be traced back to a behavioural problem. For this reason we will examine the natural behaviour of the wild rabbit in some detail.

*Crepuscular*

In most cases rabbits are described as exhibiting crepuscular behaviour venturing above ground to feed at dusk or dawn, or being completely nocturnal, only appearing in darkness. They will therefore often remain underground re-eating caecotrophs (the intermediate part-digested pellet produced and eaten directly from the anus) and sleeping during the day. Where few predators exist, rabbits will demonstrate diurnal behaviour coming out of the warren to feed during daylight hours, but this behaviour is less common. If given the chance then rabbits can be observed basking in the morning sun, a behaviour which pet rabbits will exhibit if given the chance. In captivity, many rabbits adopt a diurnal rhythm and so will be active eating foodstuffs during the day and sleeping/eating caecotrophs over night.

### Territorial

Rabbits are territorial animals, marking out their territory with their scent. Pheromones will be deposited around their territory by way of chin rubbing (from the submandibular gland), urination and the deposition of faecal pellets. Male animals will spray urine as a way of marking their territory.

Rabbits will fight with each other. As already mentioned, male animals will fight over territory. In the breeding season, female animals will also fight over nest sites.

### Prey species

Rabbits are prey species and therefore spend large amounts of their time watching for attack from foxes, stoats, weasels, mink, birds of prey and humans. This is facilitated by their laterally positioned eyes which give an almost 360° field of view as well as their excellent sense of hearing. As a prey species rabbits are particularly non-demonstrative of clinical signs of pain or discomfort, i.e. anything that would draw attention to their weakness – something which makes caring for these patients a challenge and a subject which is discussed in more detail in later sections.

Rabbits are naturally very quiet animals. They communicate with each other by thumping their hind legs on the ground as a warning when danger is near. If attacked they will scream – a blood-curdling sound to hear on a dark night.

As part of the fear response rabbits can go into a trance-like state. In some textbooks you will see mention of 'trancing' as a method of restraining rabbits for examination. By placing the rabbit on its back, it will freeze. This method is no longer advocated as an advisable way of handling rabbits as this is a stress response, resulting in physiological changes associated with fear.

### Mothering

Rabbits do not spend long with their young, only feeding them once or twice a day for a few minutes. The young are left in the burrow whilst the doe goes above ground to feed. This is important to remember if you ever try to rear orphaned rabbits as they should not be treated in the same way that pups or kittens are with respect to feeding frequency.

It is believed that the mother stimulates the kitten to urinate and defaecate, but there have been suggestions that she may not as she rarely physically grooms them and spends little time with her young.

## 1.2 Pet rabbits

As mentioned earlier, pet rabbits have descended from the fancy rabbits bred for their appearance over the last 200 years.

Traditionally, rabbits have been kept as children's pets, usually being kept singly in a hutch at the bottom of the garden. Needless to say, comparing this existence to that of the wild rabbit does lead to some questions of ethics. The rabbit is a social animal preferring to live in groups, having the freedom to move over large areas. Although not impossible, providing the space, company and stimulation for the pet rabbit can prove to be a challenge. If rabbits are allowed to run in the garden (see Fig. 1.2), then they need to be prevented from escaping. This can be difficult as they can jump, dig and squeeze through very small spaces. Their burrowing activities mean that fences must be buried to a

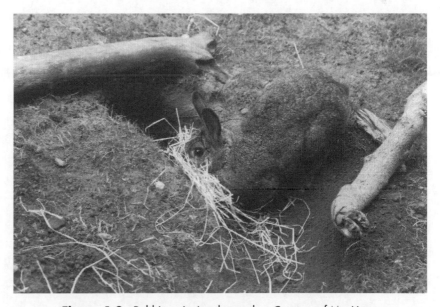

**Figure 1.2**  Rabbits enjoying the garden. Courtesy of Mrs Hare

depth of at least 30 cm to prevent escape. They also need to be protected from other animals such as cats, dogs, foxes and even birds of prey in some areas of the country. They will try to eat most things that are available, so poisonous plants need to be removed. In most cases it is easier to provide a fully enclosed wire-mesh run area, the contents of which can be controlled, rather than allowing the rabbit freedom in the garden.

### 1.2.1 House rabbits

House rabbits have become much more common over the last ten years and have probably contributed greatly to the emergence of the rabbit as the third most common pet in the UK, closely following cats and dogs.

Keeping rabbits in the house as part of the family certainly meets the requirements of company and stimulation, but it is not without its own problems. Indoor rabbits need to be toilet trained – something which in reality can prove easier in rabbits than in some dogs due to their natural behaviour outlined previously. Entire sexually mature bucks, however, will urine spray at the margins of their territory, and this is one reason for recommending routine neutering of bucks at 4–6 months of age in potential house rabbits.

Rabbits have powerful incisors and will chew anything that is in range, and therefore electric cables need to be removed from rabbit access or enclosed – to protect both the equipment and the rabbit.

If other animals are present in the house, then it may take time for them to accept each other. It is natural to assume that rabbits would be fearful of dogs or cats, but in my own experience the dog came off worse when attacked by a dominant rabbit. However, naturally both cats and dogs are potential predators of rabbits and extreme caution should be taken in introducing unfamiliar pets to house rabbits for the first time.

More information on the husbandry of house rabbits is presented in Chapter 3.

## 1.3 Breeds

The number of rabbit breeds currently recognised by the British Rabbit Council exceeds 60, and is ever increasing as new breeds are developed.

Rabbits vary hugely in their appearance from the large Flemish giant weighing around 9 kg (19.2 lb), the British giant (see Colour Plate 1) weighing 7 kg (15.2 lb), through to the Netherland dwarf (see Colour

Plate 2) weighing on average 0.9 kg (2 lb) and the Polish rabbit (see Colour Plate 3) that averages 0.75 kg (1.65 lb).

The New Zealand white is the predominant breed of the rabbit meat industry as well as the main breed of laboratory rabbit. It has been chosen for its medium-large size 4–5.5 kg (9–12 lb) and the thickness of its skin/limb structure that makes it suitable for housing on wire-floored cages.

The Angora rabbit (see Colour Plate 4) is the predominant breed of the rabbit wool industry, producing more wool per kilogram body weight than sheep at 0.2 kg wool/kg body weight/year (Okerman, 1994). The Angora rabbit's very fine long fur forms mats extremely easily and for this reason they do not make good house pets. Indeed, in the Angora wool industry they are kept without bedding material as this encourages matting of the fur.

The appearance of pet rabbits can vary somewhat to that of the wild rabbit. Although many pet rabbits such as the Dutch (see Colour Plate 5) or rex have a similar physical appearance to the wild rabbit, breeds such as the French lop (see Colour Plate 6) with large pendulous ears and foreshortened head length or Angora with copious fur have diverged from the original appearance. This has led to some associated medical problems that are discussed in Chapter 9.

Colouration of rabbits is wide and varied. They can exhibit whole colours such as white, black (see Colour Plate 7), brown (see Colour Plate 8) or patterns such as agouti or seal point (see Colour Plate 9).

More information on colours is given in Table 1.3, and some examples of rabbit breeds can be found in Table 1.4 and Colour Plates 10–12.

**Table 1.3**  Rabbit coat patterns

| Pattern | Description |
| --- | --- |
| Agouti | Light brown colouration where examination of the individual hairs shows banding – alternate light and dark areas. Agouti is the pattern found in the wild rabbit. The grey version of the agouti is the chinchilla (see Colour Plate 10) |
| Magpie | Bilaterally asymmetric colouration – this means that:<br>• One side of the face is coloured and one side is white<br>• One ear is coloured and one ear is white<br>• The feet on one side are coloured and the other side are white<br>• Over the body are stripes of colour and white<br>• The colour is usually black but could be grey or blue |
| Harlequin | Similar to magpie but the colours are orange and black (see Colour Plate 11) |
| Seal point | Extremities are darkly pigmented – ears, nose, feet and tail. Similar to a Siamese cat (see Colour Plate 9) |

**Table 1.4** Some examples of rabbit breeds

| Breed | Description |
|---|---|
| Angora | Profuse long white fluffy coat and ear tips (see Colour Plate 4) |
| Argente | Very thick short fur, erect ears |
| Belgian hare | Appearance is more like a hare than a rabbit. Long legs and ears (see Colour Plate 8) |
| British giant | Classic large white rabbit (see Colour Plate 1) |
| Chinchilla | Thick compact fur. Grey in colour similar to the rodent *Chinchilla laniger*. Erect ears (see Colour Plate 10) |
| Dutch | Black (or brown) and white face, coloured ears. Central white stripe over nose. Front half of body white, rear half black or brown (see Colour Plate 5) |
| English | White bodied with black ears, muzzle and a black stripe down the middle of the back. The body is also covered with black spots and the eyes are usually surrounded by black fur (see Colour Plate 12) |
| Himalayan | White bodied with black ears, muzzle, tail and paws (see Colour Plate 9) |
| Lionhead | Mane of fur around the face and hence the name. Generally small |
| Lop—cashmere, dwarf, English, French, German, mini | Main features are the large drooping ears and rounded nose (see Colour Plate 6) |
| Netherland dwarf | Smallest breed. Erect short ears, short fur, compact appearance (see Colour Plate 2) |
| Rex—mini or standard | Extremely short fur usually with dewlap. May be found in a variety of colours including black, blue, castor, fawn, fox, lynx, orange, otter, sable marten, sable Siamese, seal marten and seal Siamese |

## 1.4 Showing rabbits

Rabbit breeds are divided into four main groups: fancy, lops (sometimes this is included in the fancy section), normal fur and rex. Within each of these groups, rabbits are then divided up according to their colouring.

Pedigree rabbits are generally identified by a complete aluminium ring with identification numbers engraved on it, which includes the year of birth of the rabbit and an individual number unique to each rabbit. This ring is slipped over the hind leg to sit above the hock when the rabbit is young (generally before it reaches 10 weeks of age) so that as the rabbit grows the ring cannot slip off. The British Rabbit Council supplies these rings in varying sizes according to the breed of rabbit.

**Table 1.5**  Classification for showing domestic rabbit breeds

| Group | Examples of breeds |
|---|---|
| Fancy rabbits | Angora, Belgian hare, Dutch, English, lionhead |
| Lops | Mini, dwarf, English, French, German |
| Normal fur | Argente, British giant, Chinchilla, Havana |
| Rex | Blue, lilac, otter, mini |

Some examples of the rabbits found in each group are given in Table 1.5.

## Sources of further information

Rabbit Welfare Association – http://www.houserabbit.co.uk/
The British Rabbit Council – http://www.thebrc.org/
Fur and Feather magazine – http://www.furandfeather.co.uk/

## References

Moody, P.A., Cochran, V.A. and Drug, H. (1949) Serological evidence on lagomorph relationships. *Evolution* 3(1):25–33.

Okerman, L. (1994) General background. In: *Diseases of Domestic Rabbits*, 2nd edn, Blackwell Scientific Publications, Osneay Mead, Oxford, pp. 5–9.

# Anatomy and Physiology

## 2.1 Overview of anatomy and biology

Table 2.1 details some of the common biological parameters of the domestic rabbit.

## 2.2 Specific body systems

### 2.2.1 Musculoskeletal system

*Overview*

The skeletal system of rabbits is light and almost bird-like in comparison to many other terrestrial mammals. As a percentage of body weight the rabbit's skeleton is 7–8%, whereas the domestic cat's skeleton is 12–13% (Cruise and Brewer, 1994). This is further compounded by their relative muscularity with the skeletal muscles making up nearly 50% of their body weight. Rabbits are therefore extremely prone to fractures, especially of the spine and the hindlimbs due to the powerful musculature found in the rear legs and their habit of kicking out.

*Skull*

The skull is large with laterally positioned eyes giving an almost 360° view (see Colour Plate 13). The maxilla contains the usual frontal and maxillary sinuses. The mandible is slender, the temporomandibular joint

**Table 2.1** Biological parameters for the domestic rabbit *Oryctolagus cuniculus*

| Biological parameter | Average range |
|---|---|
| Body weight (kg) | 1.5–10 (dwarf Netherland – New Zealand whites and Belgian hares) |
| Rectal body temperature (°C) | 38.5–40 |
| Respiratory rate at rest (breaths/min) | 30–60 |
| Heart rate at rest (beats/min) | 130–325 (New Zealand whites – dwarf Netherland) |
| Gestation length (days) | 29–35 (average 31) |
| Litter size | 4–10 |
| Age at sexual maturity (months) Males | 5–8 |
| Females | 4–7 |
| Lifespan (years) | 6–10 |

has a wide surface area allowing considerable lateral movement of the mandible in relation to the maxilla, and the mandible is in itself narrower than the maxilla. The occipital condyles are dual in nature and both articulate with the atlas.

In the wild-type *Oryctolagus cuniculus* the head is relatively elongated with large rostral nasal passages. Overall, the head is slightly flattened from one side to the other. Inherited mandibular prognathism is common in the domestic rabbit (Huang *et al.*, 1981) as is brachycephalism (Crossley, 1995). Many of the fancy breeds of the domestic rabbit have been deliberately bred to heighten these features, resulting in more dome-shaped heads and foreshortened skull lengths (e.g. the mini lop and dwarf Netherland breeds). This can lead to problems with dental disease due to congenital malocclusion of the cheek teeth and incisors; ocular disease due to kinking of the nasolacrimal duct in the foreshortened skull and incisor root elongation which narrows the duct further; and middle ear disease due to the kinking of the Eustachian canal resulting in increased incidences of otitis media.

*Axial skeleton*

The vertebral formula of the domestic rabbit is C7, T12, L7, S4, Cy16 although 33% of rabbits have 13 thoracic vertebrae and 6 lumbar vertebrae and 23% have 13 thoracic and 7 lumbar vertebrae according to a survey performed by Greenaway *et al.* (2001).

The cervical vertebrae are box-like and small, and give overall good mobility to the neck. The thoracic vertebrae have slender and long spinous processes and give rise to the 12 paired ribs which are flattened in comparison to cat's ribs. The first pair of ribs is attached to the sternum, with pairs 8 and 9 being fused to the seventh pair. The remaining pairs of ribs (10–12) end freely in the abdominal muscles.

The thoracic vertebrae curve dorsally as they move caudally. This reaches a peak at the start of the lumbar vertebrae which have prominent slender lateral processes.

The pelvis is narrow and positioned almost vertically in the rabbit. The ilial wings are very slender and attached to the fused sacral vertebrae on the spinal column that forms the roof of the pelvis. The ilial wings meet the ischium at the acetabulum, where an accessory bone unique to rabbits called the *os acetabuli* lies. This then interposes between the ilium/ischium and the pubis. The pubis forms the floor of the pelvis and borders the obturator foramen that is oval in rabbits as compared to the cat where it is round.

### *Appendicular skeleton*

The forelimbs start proximally with the scapula. This differs from the cat in that it is slenderer and distally the scapula has a markedly hooked suprahamate process projecting caudally from the hamate process. The infraspinous fossa of the scapula is also more triangular in nature than in the cat. In cats this is much blunter. The scapula articulates with the humerus and also with a small clavicle or 'collar bone' unlike the situation in the cat. The humerus in turn articulates with the radius and ulna. In cats these two bones are separate, but in rabbits the ulna fuses to the radius in older animals and the two bones are deeply bowed. The radius and ulna articulate with the carpal bones that themselves articulate with the metacarpal bones and the five digits.

The hindlimbs start proximally with the femur. This is a long, bowed and relatively slender bone and is more rectangular in cross section, whereas in the cat it is circular, making the femur of the rabbit unsuitable for intramedullary pins when repairing fractures. The femur articulates with the tibia and fibula distally. The two bones are again fused in the rabbit. The stifle joint has a patella. The tibia articulates distally with the tarsal bones where there is a prominent calcaneous bone. The tarsal bones articulate with the metatarsal bones that articulate with the four hindlimb digits.

The hindlimbs are well muscled and powerful. Lagomorph muscle is a pale colour when viewed raw, unlike the domestic cat that is a deeper red.

## 2.2.2 Gastrointestinal system

### Oral cavity

(See also Colour Plate 14)

Dentition follows the formula I 2/1, C 0/0, Pm 3/2, M 3/3 on each side. Some of the lop breeds have one fewer maxillary cheek teeth on either side. The roots of all of the teeth are elodont in nature, that is, allowing continual growth throughout the rabbit's life. The molars' enamel is folded to provide an uneven occlusal surface with the opposite ipsilateral jaw which allows some interlocking of the teeth. Wear is kept even by the lateral movement of the mandible allowing independent left and right arcades to engage in mastication. The incisors differentiate the order Lagomorpha from Rodentia, as the rabbit, pika and hare have two smaller incisors or 'peg teeth' behind the upper two, forming an angled wedge, whereas rodents have only two upper incisors. The larger incisors have only enamel on the labial surface, whereas the smaller maxillary peg teeth have enamel on the labial and lingual sides. This allows the wedge-shaped bite plane of the incisors to form whereby the lower incisors close immediately behind the upper large incisors and fit into a groove made by the peg teeth. The permanent incisors are present at birth, although the peg teeth are replaced by permanent peg teeth around the second week of life. The deciduous premolars present at birth are replaced and joined by permanent molars by the fourth week of life. There are no canines, instead a gap or diastema exists between the incisors and premolars.

### Stomach

This is of the same form as the cat and dog, a large simple structure, with a cardiac area supplied with a strong cardiac sphincter. This makes vomiting in the rabbit virtually impossible. It is situated tucked underneath the ribcage (see Colour Plate 17). A main body or fundus and a pyloric section with a well-formed pyloric sphincter exists. The stomach wall lining contains both acid-secreting and separate pepsinogen-secreting cells. The pH of the rabbit's stomach contents is surprisingly higher than that of a cat or dog at 1.5–1.8. In addition, the stomach never truly empties in the healthy rabbit, and so an empty stomach on radiography is an abnormal finding.

## Small intestines

The first part of the small intestine is the descending duodenum that arises from the right side of the abdomen at the pyloric outflow of the stomach and moves caudally into a transverse duodenum which moves across the caudal abdomen before returning as the ascending duodenum (see Colour Plates 18 and 19). This merges into the tightly coiled jejunum, as seen in the cat and dog which then gives rise to the ileum. The total length of the small intestine in the average rabbit may be some 2–3 ft.

## The caecum and large intestines

These start at a swelling of the gut at the junction of the ileum and caecum known as the sacculus rotundus. This is infiltrated with lymphoid tissue and sits on the left dorsal aspect of the abdomen, and is a common site for foreign body impactions. From this point the caecum arises which is the first part of the gut viewed from a ventral laparotomy approach (see Colour Plates 15 and 16).

The caecum is a large, sacculated and folded organ which has three main folds in diagonal directions across the ventral aspect of the abdomen, moving first to the right flank and then back to the left. It finishes in a blind-ended thickened finger-like projection known as the vermiform appendix which is mainly lymphoid tissue. The bulk of the caecum is thin walled and possesses a semi-fluid digestive content. There is a long spiral fold along the length of the caecum.

The large intestine itself arises from an area of the ampulla (known in full as the *ampulla caecalis coli*) which sits near to the sacculus rotundus and is a smooth walled portion of the caecum with some lymphoid infiltration of its walls. The large intestine or colon is however sacculated and possesses bands of fibrous tissue running in the same plane as the gut lumen (known as taeniae) which create these sacculations (also known as haustra). The first part of the colon is known as the ascending colon and moves from the caudally located ampulla coli up to the costal arch on the ventral floor of the abdomen where it moves more dorsally and to the left. At this point the taeniae and haustra cease, and the rest of the colon forms loose coils in the dorsal part of the abdomen. It is at this point that the colon becomes known as the fusus coli, its walls becoming thickened and smooth by the large presence of nerve ganglia. These nerve cells of the enteric plexus act as a pacemaker for contraction waves in the large bowel. The distal descending colon then moves from this point, with obvious faecal pellets visible in its lumen, out through the pelvis to empty through the rectum and anus. There are a couple of anal glands just inside the anus one on either side, emptying their secretions onto the faecal pellets.

### Physiology of large intestine function

In the rabbit there are two types of faecal pellet produced. One is a true faecal pellet, comprising waste material in a dry and light brown spherical form. The other is a much darker, mucus covered pellet known as a caecotroph. This latter pellet is the one eaten directly from the anus, by the rabbit, as soon as it is produced. In the wild these caecotrophs are more commonly produced during the middle of the day when the rabbit is often underground. In captivity they are often produced over night, but may be produced at any time. The caecotroph contains plant material from which all of the nutrients have yet to be extracted, hence the second pass through the digestive system. Research has shown that the caecotrophs have a higher protein, lower fibre (on a dry matter basis) and higher water content than true faeces (Sakaguchi, 2003).

The selection of material to form the caecotroph is performed by the large bowel under the controlling influence of the nerve ganglia in the fusus coli. Once food has passed through the small intestine, it accumulates in the proximal colon, contained in the multiple haustra. At this point the proximal colon produces a reverse peristaltic wave that flushes the fine particulate matter into the caecum. Here microbial fermentation occurs, helping to break down the tough cellulose and hemicellulose walls of the plant material. The larger fibre particles which cannot be digested adequately in the caecum are selected out by the proximal colon for passage out of the gut and into the caecotroph pellet which will be re-eaten directly from the rabbit's anus, and so achieve a second digestion process. These caecotrophs are covered in mucus to protect their microbial contents from some of the onslaught of the acidic stomach contents, so allowing further microbial breakdown of the fibre. The smaller fibre particles which were flushed back into the caecum, once broken down as far as possible, will be then passed out of the caecum, back into the colon, and excreted as the true dry faecal pellet which is not re-eaten.

### Liver

The rabbit liver has four lobes. There is a gall bladder, which has a separate opening from the pancreatic duct into the proximal duodenum (see Colour Plate 18). The main bile pigment is biliverdin, rather than the more usual bilirubin seen in cats and dogs. This has an implication for the biochemical tests employed in detecting liver disease in rabbits as serum total bilirubin measurement is not a useful indicator of liver function in the rabbit. Indeed, there is not one specific test for liver function/disease in rabbits. The measurement of alanine aminotransferase and aspartate aminotransferase has been recorded for liver damage assessment although neither is liver specific. Alkaline phosphatase elevations in rabbits are more likely to be due to intestinal damage, rather than hepatic damage. The measurement of bile acid levels has recently been shown to be a useful indicator of remaining liver functional mass.

### Pancreas

This is a diffuse organ, suspended in the loop of the duodenum. There is one single pancreatic duct, separate from the bile duct, emptying into the proximal duodenum.

## 2.2.3 Respiratory system

### Upper respiratory tract

The paired nostrils can be closed tightly shut in lagomorphs. They communicate caudally with a large nasal passage. Rabbits like horses are nasal breathers, with the nasopharynx permanently locked around the epiglottis; hence, upper respiratory disease or evidence of mouth breathing is a poor sign. The nasolacrimal ducts open onto the rostral floor of the nasal passages as with other mammals.

The epiglottis is not visible easily from the oral cavity, making direct intubation difficult. It is narrow and elongated and leads into the larynx, which has limited vocal fold development, hence the lack of frequent vocalization in the rabbit. The larynx leads into the trachea that has incomplete C-shaped cartilage rings for support.

*Lower respiratory tract*

The trachea bifurcates into two primary bronchi. There are two lungs, which are relatively small in proportion to the overall rabbit's body size. This means that even small amounts of lung damage can lead to problems. This also means that the majority of the inspiratory effort comes from the movement of the diaphragm and abdominal musculature rather than the intercostal muscles and rib cage movement. Each lung has three lobes, with the cranial ones being the smallest (see Colour Plates 19 and 20).

*Respiratory physiology*

As mentioned, much of the impetus for inspiration derives from the muscular contraction and flattening of the diaphragm (see Colour Plate 20). The stimulus for this is much the same as for cats and dogs with a decrease in oxygen within the blood being detected by chemoreceptors inside the carotid bodies and an increase in carbon dioxide and hydrogen ions being detected in the medulla, causing an increase in the depth and rate of respiration. In rabbits though, we know that the lungs are also the 'shock organ'. In cats and dogs the gut is the 'shock organ' meaning that when acutely damaged or traumatised anaphylactic chemicals are released and pooling of blood occurs within the gastrointestinal system so accelerating the shock process. In rabbits, it appears that the lung parenchyma possesses a cellular population well supplied with anaphylactic mediating chemicals, strong enough to cause fluid extravasation and blood pooling as well as spasms within the walls of the main pulmonary arterial supply that can lead to rapid right-sided heart failure. This is of particular importance when performing chest surgery and when attempting to anaesthetise a rabbit.

The average respiratory rate in rabbits ranges from 30 to 60 breaths per minute at rest.

## 2.2.4 Cardiovascular system

*Heart*

The heart in rabbits is relatively small in relation to body size (see Colour Plate 20). It differs from cats and dogs in that the right atrioventricular valve has only two cusps instead of three. In addition, as mentioned above, the pulmonary artery has a large amount of smooth muscle in its wall that can contract vigorously during anaphylactic shock, causing immediate right-sided cardiac overload and failure.

### Arteries and veins

Most of the vascular layout is similar to that seen in cats and dogs. One or two access sites are worthy of mention though. As far as peripheral veins for blood sampling and catheter placement are concerned, the following list (Table 2.2) may be useful.

The eye has also a large venous plexus at the medial canthus, draining the orbit. This is an important structure to avoid when enucleating the eye or operating periorbitally.

## 2.2.5 Lymphatic system

### Spleen

The spleen is a flattened structure, oblong in nature and attached to the greater curvature of the stomach, and is thus found predominantly on the left side. There are the usual white and red pulp areas within the structure of the spleen as found in cats and dogs.

### Thymus

The thymus is a large structure in the cranial thoracic compartment even in the adult rabbit as it does not disappear with age. It has the same functions as for any other mammal in that it provides the body with the T-cell population of lymphocytes.

### Lymph nodes

The root of the mesentery supporting the digestive tract is well supplied with lymph nodes, as is the hilar area of the lungs where the two main bronchi diverge to supply each lung. In addition there are superficial lymph nodes in the popliteal, prescapular and submandibular areas, although these are much smaller deposits than are found in dogs and cats, and so often go unnoticed except when diseased.

**Table 2.2** Vessels for sampling and intravenous fluid administration

| Vessel | Position | Access for catheterisation/ sampling |
|---|---|---|
| Lateral ear vein | This runs, as its name suggests, along the lateral margin of either ear | It may be entered using a 25- or 27-gauge needle/catheter and used for slow intravenous injections and blood sampling. Application of local anaesthetic cream to the area 2–3 minutes prior to venipuncture is recommended to avoid the rabbit jumping at the critical moment and to encourage vasodilation |
| Central ear artery | This runs along the midline of the outer aspect of each pinna | It is a large vessel and is generally avoided for blood sampling due to fear of thrombus formation, which would cut off the blood supply to the ear tip, leading to avascular necrosis. It may however be used in an emergency with care using a 25- to 27-gauge needle and applying pressure to the vessel once sampled. It is not advised for intravenous fluid administration |
| Cephalic vein | This runs in a similar position to that seen in cats and dogs on the antebrachium | It may be split into two in some individuals, but may be used for intravenous fluids and sampling. 25- to 27-gauge catheters may be used |
| Jugular veins | These are prominent in the rabbit and run in a 'V' shape from the manubrium of the sternum to the base of each respective ear | Their use should be carefully considered though as they form the major part of the drainage of blood from the orbit of the eye. Therefore, if a haematoma and thrombus forms and blocks the lumen of a jugular vein, severe orbital oedema may occur, with possible damaging effects. Blood sampling may be performed using a 23- to 25-gauge needle and 2 mL syringe. It is possible to catheterise a jugular vein in an emergency to delivery intravenous fluid therapy, but a cut-down technique generally is required. 23- to 25-gauge catheters may be used for this purpose |
| Saphenous vein | This runs across the lateral aspect of the hock as in cats and dogs | 25- to 27-gauge catheters may be used to cannulate this vessel for fluid therapy. A blood sample may also be collected from this vein with patience |

## 2.2.6 Haematological system

### Morphology of blood cells

The blood cells of the rabbit are essentially like those of the cat or dog. There is a difference in the staining of the rabbit neutrophil though that often resembles the cat or dog eosinophil. For this reason the rabbit neutrophil is often known as the 'pseudoeosinophil'. Many rabbits have more lymphocytes than pseudoeosinophils, resembling other mammals such as cattle, rather than cats and dogs where the neutrophil is the commonest white blood cell.

In other respects the red and white cell morphology of the rabbit resembles those of the domestic cat and dog.

### Blood cell counts

The quoted ranges for red cells have been questioned for the domestic rabbit as Harcourt-Brown and Baker (2001) have suggested that the typical packed cell volume should be between 30 and 40%, with values exceeding 45% suggesting dehydration and values less than 30% indicating anaemia. See Table 2.3 for normal haematological values for the domestic rabbit.

The white cell counts may also be used to predict disease as the alteration in the ratio of neutrophils to lymphocytes and overall cell numbers has been shown to be associated with disease (Hinton *et al.*, 1982).

**Table 2.3**  Haematological values for a normal healthy domestic rabbit

| Parameter | Value |
|---|---|
| Red blood cell count | $5.1–7.9 \times 10^{12}/L$ |
| Packed cell volume | 33–50% |
| Haemoglobin | 10–17.4 g/dL |
| Mean cell volume | 57.8–66.5 fL |
| Mean cell haemoglobin | 17.1–23.5 pg |
| Mean cell haemoglobin concentration | 29–37 g/dL |
| Platelets | $250–650 \times 10^9/L$ |
| White cell count | $5.2–12.5 \times 10^9/L$ |
| Neutrophils | 30–50% |
| Lymphocytes | 30–60% |
| Eosinophils | 0–5% |
| Basophils | 0–8% |
| Monocytes | 2–10% |

Adapted from Mader (2003) and Gillett (1994). L, litre; g, gram; dL, decalitre; fL, femtolitre; pg, picogram.

In addition, the neutrophil to lymphocyte ratio has also been suggested as a useful indicator of disease (McLaughlin and Fish, 1994). However, things are not so straight forward as the ratio of neutrophil to lymphocyte varies with age, changing from 33:60 at 2 months of age to 45:45 once over 1 year of age in healthy rabbits (Jain, 1986).

Changes in the white cell counts and ratios that have been associated with stress include a mature neutrophilia with a lymphopaenia and an increase in plasma cortisol (Toth and January, 1990).

An eosinophilia has been associated with intestinal parasitism as well as traumatic wound healing (Fudge, 2000).

Basophil counts may be higher than suggested in Table 2.3 and the rabbit can still be clinically healthy in one study (Benson and Paul-Murphy, 1999).

A monocytosis may indicate chronic disease but normal monocyte counts have also been found in the presence of chronic disease (Harcourt-Brown, 2002).

## 2.2.7 Urinary system

### Kidneys

The kidneys are similar in shape to the cat's kidneys as the classical bean shape (see Colour Plate 21). Unlike the cat they are unipapillate, i.e. all of the collecting ducts converge to one point. The right kidney is slightly more cranial to the left, and they are often separated from the ventral lumbar spine by large fat deposits in many domestic rabbits. A single ureter arises from each kidney and traverses across the abdominal cavity to empty into the urinary bladder.

The microscopic structure of the kidneys is much the same as that for cats and dogs with the above exception. Physiologically, rabbit urine often contains large amounts of calcium unlike many other domestic species.

### Bladder

The urinary bladder is functionally and anatomically similar to that seen in cats and dogs (see Colour Plate 22). The lining is composed of transitional cell epithelium. The urethra in the male rabbit exits through the pelvis and out through the penis. In females the urethra opens onto the floor of the vagina, which passes through the pelvis and out through the vulva.

**Table 2.4**  Urinalysis results for a normal domestic rabbit

| Parameter | Value in a healthy domestic rabbit |
|---|---|
| Urine volume | 10–35 mL/kg/day average (depending on diet) |
| Urine specific gravity | 1.003–1.036 |
| Urine erythrocyte numbers | <5 erythrocytes per high power field |
| Urine protein levels | Trace to absent (may be more in juveniles) |
| Urine colour | Varies from pale yellow to deep red depending on presence/absence of porphyrins |
| Urine average pH | 8.2 |
| Urine crystals | Small volumes of ammonium magnesium phosphate or calcium carbonate are normal |

### Urinary physiology

Like most herbivores, rabbits' urine is alkaline in nature, with a pH varying between 6.5 and 8. The pH will become acidic if the rabbit has been anorectic for 24 hours or more. Commonly in many domestic rabbits, the urine will contain varying amounts of calcium carbonate. This is because of the rabbit's unique method of calcium metabolism. Here, unlike cats, dogs, humans, etc., whereby some down-regulation of calcium absorption will occur at the gut if body levels of calcium are high, in the rabbit the gut just absorbs as much calcium as possible at all times. This means that any excess calcium needs to be excreted by the kidneys into the urine, where crystals of calcium carbonate frequently form owing to the alkaline nature of the urine. This can be seen as tan-coloured silt in the urine excreted. In addition, other pigments may be seen in rabbits' urine, known as porphyrins. These are plant pigments contained in the food consumed, and these are excreted in the urine, making it appear anywhere from a dark yellow colour to a deep wine red colour. This may mimic haematuria; therefore, to diagnose blood in the urine it is often necessary to examine the urine produced microscopically. A positive diagnosis is made when >5 red blood cells per high power field are seen. See Table 2.4 for normal urinalysis results for the domestic rabbit.

## 2.2.8 Reproductive system

### Male (buck's) reproductive system

The paired testes can move from an inguinal position within the thin-skinned scrotal sacs to an intra-abdominal position through the open inguinal canal (see Colour Plate 22). The scrotal sacs are sparsely haired and lie on either side of the anogenital area.

Each testicle has the usual epididymal structure comprising the convoluted chambers of the vas deferens where the spermatozoa mature. The vas deferens passes up the scrotal cord into the abdomen before angling caudally to pass through the pelvic cavity and join the single urethra. Here a series of secondary reproductive organs are attached and empty. The glands which are found in the buck are a dorsal and a smaller ventral prostate which are bilobed. In addition there is a bilobed vesicular gland, a bilobed coagulating gland and a bilobed bulbo-urethral gland. The urethra then passes out of the pelvis and enters the penis. In the buck this is a short structure and projects ventrally and caudally. There is no evidence of an os penis or of a glans penis as is found in the dog. The prepuce itself has numerous small preputial glands in the dermis, and there are a couple of inguinal glands situated either side of the penis which secrete a brown sebum clearly seen adjacent to the anus.

### Female (doe's) reproductive system

The ovaries are small elongated bean-shaped structures, supported by the ovarian ligament and lying just caudal to each respective kidney. The ovarian artery often splits into two parts after leaving the aorta, and it along with the rest of the reproductive tract is frequently encased in large amounts of fat, forming a fat deposition site.

The form of the doe's reproductive tract is known as a duplex uterus. This is because, unlike the cat and the dog, there is no common body to the uterus. Rather there are effectively two separate uteri with separate cervices emptying into the vagina. The vagina is large and thin walled with the urethra opening onto its floor cranial to the pelvis. The vulva therefore is a common opening for the reproductive and urinary systems as with cats and dogs and unlike many rodents. The vulva lies just cranial to the anus and is flanked on either side by the inguinal glands as with the buck.

The doe has on average four pairs of mammary glands, extending from the inguinal region up to the axillary areas.

## 2.2.9 Reproductive physiology

### Male (buck) rabbit

The usual hormones found in cats and dogs are believed to be responsible for spermatogenesis in the buck. Sertoli cells in the testes are acted upon by follicle-stimulating hormone (FSH) from the anterior pituitary to produce oestrogens and encourage spermatozoan development. Leydig cells are found in the parenchyma and are acted upon by luteinising hormone (LH) from the anterior pituitary to produce testosterone to encourage secondary male characteristics and behaviour. The fluctuations of these hormones are on a very seasonal time clock triggered by the lengthening daylight encountered in the spring. This is mediated through the pineal gland in the brain which has links from the eyes, and controls the hormone melatonin which in turn controls the pituitary release of FSH and LH.

### Female (doe) rabbit

The hormone hierarchy is much the same for does as it is for cats and dogs, with FSH stimulating follicle development and LH the development of the corpus luteum. Rabbits are like cats in that they are induced ovulators. Waves of follicles swell and regress during the course of the season, starting to increase in activity in early spring. If not mated these follicles will often dominate the cycle for 12–16 days at a time. In fact, there is no real anoestrus phase in does, and they merely experience a slight waning in activity for 1–2 days and then go back into 'heat' again. During peak sexual activity the vulva is often deeply congested and almost purple in colour and considerably enlarged.

Once mated the male's semen may form a copulatory plug which is a gelatinous accumulation of sperm which drops out of the doe's vagina 4–6 hours post-mating. Gestation lasts from 29 to 35 days, with the foetus forming a haemochorial placenta (where the outer chorion layer of the foetal placental membrane burrows into the lining of the uterus so that it directly attaches to the blood in the intrauterine vessels) at about day 13. This is a common time for abortions to occur. A pregnant doe will often remove fur from her ventrum to line the nest in the latter few days prior to parturition.

Parturition itself is rarely difficult, with dystocia being uncommon. The doe only nurses the kittens once a day for 20 minutes or so, often in the early morning. It is therefore not uncommon for owners to think that the doe is neglecting her young, as she will often spend the rest of the time eating and away from the litter.

Pseudopregnancy or phantom pregnancy is not uncommon. This generally occurs after unsuccessful mating by a buck or repeated mounting by another doe. A corpus luteum forms and this lasts for 15–17 days during which the doe may produce milk, and nest build. At this time the doe is frequently susceptible to mastitis.

## 2.2.10 Endocrine system

### Pituitary gland

This is situated at the base of the brain and is responsible as in other mammals for controlling a number of other endocrine glands such as the adrenal glands and the reproductive organs. As with other mammals there are both a posterior and an anterior pituitary gland. Principle hormones produced by the anterior pituitary gland include FSH and LH which directly affect the testes/ovaries. Also, prolactin (which affects amongst other things milk production in the lactating doe), growth hormone, thyroid-stimulating hormone (which as its name suggests acts on the thyroid gland) and adrenocorticotropic hormone (which acts on the adrenal gland to increase secretions) are all produced by the anterior pituitary gland. The posterior pituitary gland is responsible for producing antidiuretic hormone (also known as vasopressin which encourages water retention in the kidneys) and oxytocin (which stimulates milk let-down in the lactating doe and uterine contractions).

### Adrenal glands

These are paired as with other mammals and situated medial to their respective kidney and closely associated with the major blood vessels of the abdomen (see Colour Plate 21). They are responsible for producing adrenaline and associated hormones in the medulla of the gland which are under neurological control mainly and responsible for some of the responses to fright and flight reflexes.

The cortex produces glucocorticoids such as cortisol and corticosterone under the influence of adreno corticotropic hormone from the pituitary gland and a mineralocorticoid (aldosterone). Finally, a series of reproductive hormones are secreted such as androstenedione by the adrenal glands.

### Thyroid and parathyroid glands

The thyroid gland in the rabbit is situated in the neck closely associated with the trachea and the smaller parathyroid glands. The thyroid gland is responsible for producing thyroxine (T4) and tri-iodothyronine

(T3) under the influence of thyroid-stimulating hormone from the pituitary gland. The principle hormone is T4 and this regulates a number of systemic processes associated with growth.

The parathyroid glands are often closely associated with the thyroid glands and are responsible for regulating the body calcium levels via two hormones: calcitonin (which decreases plasma calcium levels) and parathyroid hormone (which increases plasma calcium levels).

### Pancreas

The endocrine pancreas in rabbits is similar to that in other mammals with islets of Langerhans possessing beta cells that secrete insulin (that reduces blood glucose levels) and alpha cells which secrete glucagons (that increase blood glucose levels). The rabbit has been rarely diagnosed with diabetes mellitus as with most herbivorous animals it can withstand the absence of insulin more readily than carnivorous species (Bentley, 1998).

## 2.2.11 Skin

The skin structure of the rabbit is similar to that found in the cat and dog. There are some variations, with breeds such as the lops having extra skin folds as 'dewlaps' around the neck region ventrally, particularly in does. In addition, such extra folds of skin may be found around the anogenital area leading to increased risk of urine and faecal soiling.

Rabbits do not have foot pads as seen in cats and dogs. Instead they have thick fur covering the toes and metatarsal areas that are pressed flat to the ground.

In addition to the para-anal scent glands mentioned above, there are a series of discrete submandibular chin glands. These are used as in cats to mark territory and also, in the case of does, to mark their young to distinguish them from others.

The rabbit has no skin sweat glands except a few along the margins of the lips. This means that they are prone to heat stress relatively easily at temperatures greater than 28°C.

The presence of many vibrissae or sensitive hairs around the lips and chin is important, as rabbits cannot see anything immediately below their mouths, and so rely on touch to manipulate food towards the mouth.

## 2.2.12 Nervous system and eyes

*Eyes*

Rabbits have very prominent eyes, which allow a near 360° field of vision, which is necessary to detect potential predators (see Colour Plate 13). There is a prominent third eyelid that moves from the medial canthus of the eye and often has a large amount of lymphoid reactive tissue within its structure as well as possessing both a deep and superficial tear gland. The deep gland is also often referred to as the Harderian gland and is often enlarged in the buck during the breeding season and possesses two lobes in both the sexes. In addition, there are four other lacrimal glands in the rabbit.

There are two blind spots due to the lateral position of the rabbit's eyes: just in front of the rabbit below the mouth and immediately behind the head. The former means that the rabbit detects its food at close range by smell and by 'touch' with the sensitive whiskers known as vibrissae which fringe the lips.

There is only one ventrally situated lacrimal puncta to drain tears from the periocular area. This immediately enters a small lacuna or swelling before entering the nasolacrimal duct properly which passes through the lacrimal and maxillary bones before looping around the roots of the maxillary incisors to empty in the rostral nasal passage.

*Nervous system*

The brain is organised in a similar fashion to other mammals. It is covered by the meninges from external to internal layers: the dura mater, the arachnoid mater and the pia mater. The main difference in the visual appearance of the rabbit brain from that of the dog, for example, is its lack of obvious surface gyri or folds (see Colour Plate 23). Rather the rabbit brain surface appears smooth.

Rabbits possess the same 12 cranial nerves as other higher vertebrates. The main problem with assessing neurological function in rabbits is their lack of response to many noxious stimuli as part of the fear or freezing response. This of course does not mean that they appreciate pain less than other mammals, rather their demonstration of pain perception is different.

The fragile spinal column means spinal cord damage is a common traumatic injury to rabbits. In addition, vestibular disease due to otitis media/interna and stimulation of the vestibulocochlear (VIII cranial nerve) is another common neurological disease of rabbits.

The autonomic nervous system to the gastrointestinal tract, particularly the caecum and colon, is very well developed and centred on the fusus coli section of the colon (see subsection 2.2.2).

# References

Benson, K.G. and Paul-Murphy, J. (1999) Clinical pathology of the domestic rabbit. *Veterinary Clinics of North America: Exotic Animal Practice* 2:539–552.

Bentley, P.J. (1998) *Comparative Vertebrate Endocrinology*, 3rd edn, Cambridge University Press, Cambridge.

Crossley, D.A. (1995) Clinical aspects of lagomorph dental anatomy: the rabbit (*Oryctolagus cuniculus*). *Journal of Veterinary Dentistry* 12:137–140.

Cruise, L.J. and Brewer, N.R. (1994) Anatomy. In: *The Biology of the Laboratory Rabbit*, 2nd edn (eds, Manning, P.J., Ringler, D.H. and Newcomer, C.E.), Academic Press, San Diego, pp. 47–61.

Fudge, A.M. (2000) Rabbit hematology. In: *Laboratory Medicine: Avian and Exotic Pets* (ed., Fudge, A.M.), W.B. Saunders, Philadelphia, pp. 273–275.

Gillett, G.S. (1994) Selected drug dosages and clinical reference data. In: *The Biology of the Laboratory Rabbit*, 2nd edn (eds, Manning, P.J., Ringler, D.H. and Newcomer, C.E.), Academic Press, San Diego, pp. 467–472.

Greenaway, J.B., Partlow, G.D. and Gonsholt, N.L. (2001) Anatomy of the lumbosacral spinal cord in rabbits. *Journal of the American Animal Hospital Association* 37:27–34.

Harcourt-Brown, F.M. (2002) Clinical pathology. In: *Textbook of Rabbit Medicine*, Elsevier Science Ltd, Oxford, pp. 140–164.

Harcourt-Brown, F.M. and Baker, S.J. (2001) Parathyroid hormone, haematological and biochemical parameters in relation to dental disease and husbandry in pet rabbits. *Journal of Small Animal Practice* 42:130–136.

Hinton, M., Jones, D.R.E. and Festing, M.F.W. (1982) Haematological findings in healthy and diseased rabbits, a multivariate analysis. *Laboratory Animals* 16:123–129.

Huang, C.M., Mi, M.P. and Vogt, D.W. (1981) Mandibular prognathism in the rabbit: discrimination between single locus and multifactorial modes of inheritance. *Journal of Heredity* 72:296–298.

Jain, N.C. (1986) Haematology of laboratory and miscellaneous animals. In: *Schalm's Veterinary Hematology*, 4th edn, Lea and Febiger, Philadelphia, pp. 276–282.

Mader, D. (2003) Basic approach to veterinary care. In: *Ferrets, Rabbits and Rodents: Clinical Medicine and Surgery*, 2nd edn (eds, Quesenberry, K.E. and Carpenter, J.W.), Elsevier Saunders, St Louis, Missouri, pp. 147–154.

McLaughlin, R.M. and Fish, R.E. (1994) Clinical biochemistry and haematology. In: *The Biology of the Laboratory Rabbit*, 2nd edn (eds, Manning, P.J., Ringler, D.H. and Newcomer, C.E.), Academic Press, London, pp. 111–124.

Sakaguchi, E. (2003) Digestive strategies of small hindgut fermenters. *Animal Science Journal* 74:327–337.

Toth, L.A. and January, B. (1990) Physiological stabilization of rabbits after shipping. *Laboratory Animal Science* 40:384–387.

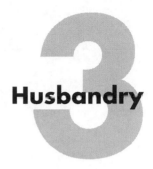

# Husbandry

Wild rabbits are social animals, living in groups of between two and eight. Historically, pet rabbits were kept as individual animals. However, in recent years this is becoming less common, with outside rabbits kept in pairs or even groups and the increasing numbers of rabbits being kept as house pets. Although it is easy to think that rabbits will be happier kept in groups, you should remember that some rabbits will fight, especially males kept in the same area and rabbits newly introduced to each other.

In the following section discussion is aimed at pet rabbits. However, you should remember that rabbits are used in research and are farmed for meat. Therefore, the way in which rabbits are looked after is regulated by Home Office regulations, government code of conduct for husbandry of laboratory rabbits (Home Office, 2003) and farmed rabbits (DEFRA, 2008).

Although many aspects of husbandry such as nutrition will be similar for both outside and house rabbits, the following sections examine hutch rabbits and house rabbits separately.

## 3.1 Hutch rabbits

As the name suggests hutch rabbits are predominantly kept outside in some form of a hutch. This, however, does not exclude them from having access to the garden or even the house – just that they spend most of their time outside.

## 3.1.1 Housing

The best hutch should have the following features:

- Raised off the ground
- Separate run and nest area
- Situated in an area out of direct sun
- Constructed from a material that can be cleaned
- Escape proof
- Waterproof

The hutch (see Fig. 3.1) should obviously be of a size that allows the rabbit to move about freely. Various different guidelines for the minimum space requirements can be found. The minimum length of accommodation should be 1.5 m (RSPCA, 2003) or allow three hops from end to end (Meredith and Crossley, 2002). The width should be 0.6 m (RSPCA, 2003) with a height of 0.45 m according to DEFRA (2008) or 0.75 m according to the RSPCA (2003). Other authors dictate a height sufficient to allow the rabbit to sit up with ears erect (Mullan and Main, 2006). Minimum floor space requirements vary from 0.54 (Home Office guidelines) to 0.56 m$^2$ (DEFRA, 2008).

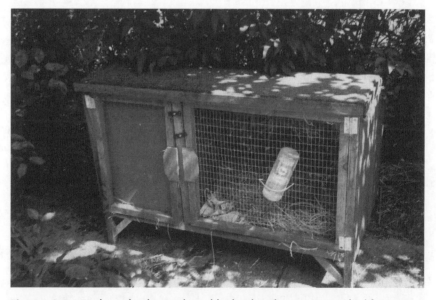

**Figure 3.1**   Traditional style wooden rabbit hutch with part wire-meshed front. Note sip feeder water bottle.

A study of rabbit owners (Mullan and Main, 2006) found that the average hutch size was smaller than the recommended guidelines at 1.16 m long, 0.58 m wide. If a rabbit has access to an outside run then this may be acceptable; however, if a rabbit spends most if its time in the hutch or if more than one rabbit is kept there then they obviously need more space. The size also depends on the breed of rabbit being kept. The dimensions will obviously differ between those required for a Netherland Dwarf and a Flemish giant.

Many hutches are home made and whilst owners may have the best of intentions they may not be aware of these guidelines. Owner education should preferably therefore start before the rabbit is bought, providing information about the housing requirements.

Hutches should have a solid area where the rabbit can make a nest and a meshed run area. The nest area should contain straw and/or hay so that the rabbit can make a bed. The run area needs to allow adequate ventilation to prevent respiratory disease, but also provide enough shelter from rain, snow and wind if outside. If mesh or chicken wire is used then the mesh should be small enough to prevent birds and vermin from entering the run – rabbit food can be attractive to other species.

The siting of the hutch in the garden is important for this reason also. Whilst it is easy to think of having the hutch in one position in the garden, sometimes it is more sensible to move the hutch according to the time of year. During the summer ensure that the hutch is not in direct sunlight as it can be surprising just how hot a wooden hutch can get. In the winter it may be necessary to move the hutch to a sheltered area of the garden or even a shed or garage to protect it from bad weather. If weather is particularly bad and shelter is not available then covering the wire mesh front with a Hessian sack can be carried out to provide shelter. This should be removed once the worst of the weather has passed as it will restrict airflow through the hutch and could lead to possible respiratory problems.

As mentioned above, extremes of temperature are a possibility. Many hutches especially those that are home made have a waterproof roof covering made of bitumen. This absorbs heat in the summer, increasing the temperature with the hutch. Rabbits cannot sweat or pant and can only maintain their body temperature through behaviour and location. Temperatures in excess of 25°C can prove fatal. If they are unable to find a cooler area then hyperthermia is a distinct possibility.

Most bought and home-made hutches are made of wood, which has obvious problems – wood can be chewed, urine can soak into the wood causing it to rot and can be difficult to clean fully.

### 3.1.2 Flooring/bedding

The floor of most hutches is made of wood. This needs to be smooth to avoid splinters. The wood should not be painted or varnished as rabbits will chew this and remove the paint. Urine will soak into the wood so some sort of absorbent material such as wood shavings or sawdust needs to be put down in the run area and hay or straw in the bedding area. This needs to be cleaned regularly to reduce soaking of the wood.

The floor should not be too abrasive so as to prevent trauma of the hocks. Sore hocks in rabbits can also develop due to the rabbit being overweight or as a consequence of neurological/spinal problems resulting in a plantigrade stance placing pressure on the hocks rather than the feet. Any damage to the skin of the hocks can be difficult to treat so should be prevented wherever possible.

Within the secluded bedding area, hay and straw are the best materials to use as these are warm and can be used to build a nest as well as being safe to eat.

### 3.1.3 Food/water provision

Fresh food and water needs to be available for the rabbit at all times. In the wild, rabbits will spend a large amount of their time grazing and this should be replicated in captivity wherever possible. Feeding rabbits concentrated foods provides them with large amounts of energy and these foods should not be available all day and every day, otherwise the rabbit can end up obese as well as leading to poor dental wear of the teeth, resulting in dental disease.

Instead fibre should be provided *ad libitum* in the form of fresh grass, good quality hay or dried grass, supported with fresh leafy vegetables such as kale, spring greens, herb lettuces such as romaine, lambs leaf, etc., and a small amount of concentrate and root vegetables such as carrots. Pelleted concentrates are preferable to a dry mix as rabbits will select their favorite foodstuffs from the mix, and therefore consume an unbalanced diet. A homogenous pelleted feed therefore removes this choice.

Water is usually provided in a water bottle with a sip feeder. Positioning of this is important to ensure that the rabbit can reach the tip. Positioning the bottle too low down will make drinking difficult and too high obviously means that the rabbit will not be able to reach it. Fresh water should be provided daily. The water bottle should also be observed for leaks as older bottles have a tendency to drip leading to soaking bedding and possible lack of a water supply for the rabbit. Bottles should be cleaned with a bottle cleaner rather than just rinsing as algae can build up inside them.

Although bottles are the commonest method of providing water, rabbits can drink out of a bowl and some rabbits prefer this. In a veterinary hospital basis it is best to enquire of the owner which type of water feeder the rabbit prefers and if in doubt then provide both.

Bowls should be made of a material that cannot be chewed and can be easily cleaned. Ceramic or metal is preferable to plastic. Also, the bowls need to be positioned so that they cannot be knocked over by rabbits jumping around the cage. Ceramic bowls are heavier and therefore less likely to be knocked over. However, a stand can be used to hold the bowls and may be preferable as it reduces the amount of bedding contamination.

### 3.1.4 Cleaning the hutch

The hutch needs to be kept clean to prevent environmental microbial build-up and potential disease situations as well as reducing damp or sodden bedding which can lead to skin maceration and infections. In addition, ammonia build-up from bacterial degradation of urine and faeces leads to damage to the respiratory tract and facilitates respiratory tract infections. The size or availability of an attached run will determine how much time the rabbit spends in its hutch and therefore will influence how frequently the hutch will need to be cleaned out.

Most rabbits will select an area of the hutch to use as the main toilet area, so this area can be cleaned out more frequently. Nest areas are usually kept fairly clean and do not require to be cleaned out as often as the run area, but this is highly dependent on how big the hutch is in the first place. Too small a hutch or cage will lead to soiling of nest material and food/water bowls and so requires more regular cleaning.

The entire hutch should be cleaned out once to twice a week, removing all of the soiled material. If a run area is available then rabbits can be placed here whilst cleaning is taking place. If the run is dry then removing material and replacing substrate will be sufficient. However, cleaning of the floor with a disinfectant should also take place. It is important when using this to ensure that the floor is allowed to dry out completely before replacing substrate and returning the rabbit to the hutch.

Disinfectants should be used with caution. There are several animal-friendly disinfectants currently available, and where possible these should be used in preference to household detergents such as bleach which can give off toxic fumes as well as being highly corrosive and irritant if they come into contact with the skin. See section 3.4 for further information on disinfectants.

### 3.1.5 Run area

Exercise is important and a run area or access to the garden should be allowed wherever possible. However, it is important that this run area can both prevent the rabbit from escaping and protect the rabbit from predators. Providing a run area for one or more rabbits requires a great deal of preparation. Mesh wire should be either laid on the ground or buried under the ground to a depth of at least 0.4 m in order to prevent burrowing. Height-wise the surrounding fence needs to be high enough to prevent the rabbit from jumping out if startled. If foxes are around then the run should also prevent them from entering; therefore, covering the run area may also be required. It is also advisable to prevent pet rabbits from coming in contact with wild rabbits due to the dangers of myxomatosis which is transmitted via the rabbit flea *Spilopsyllus cuniculi*. Following all of this you may decide that it is easier to keep the rabbit in the hutch. However, allowing the rabbit access to an outside run allows them to demonstrate more natural behaviour such as basking, and allows them to exercise. It also may help with wearing down of claws especially if the rabbit has access to rough ground or a paved area.

Within the run area a variety of plants can be provided for the rabbit, but it is important to make sure that no species of plant poisonous to rabbits such as lupins or foxgloves, for example, can be eaten. See Appendix 2 for a list of common garden poisonous plants.

If a run area to allow exercise is not possible, there are currently several varieties of rabbit harness available commercially which allow the owner to walk their rabbit (see Fig. 3.2). Care should be taken to use the correct harness as properly fitting ones prevent damage to the neck and back. Care should also be taken to ensure that the harness is correctly secured and does not come undone (see Fig. 3.3). Owners also need to ensure that the rabbit is fully vaccinated and that areas where dogs are walked are avoided.

### 3.1.6 Grouping of rabbits

Rabbits are social creatures and small groups or at least pairs of rabbits seem to be more content in a domestic situation. Care should be taken to ensure any mixing of potential cage mates is performed at as young an

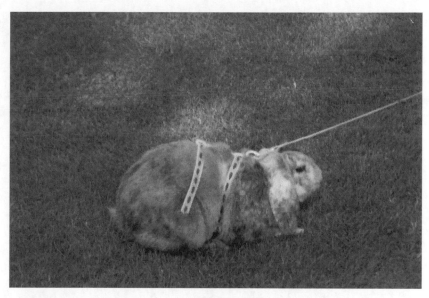

**Figure 3.2** Typical rabbit harness with leash allowing 'walking' of rabbits for exercise.

age as possible to minimise the risks of fighting and rejection. Males and females can be kept together providing the males are neutered (assuming no kittens are wanted). It is also advisable to neuter does on health grounds to prevent uterine cancers.

Females can of course be kept together as a single sex group and similar males may be kept as a single sex group, although again neutering is advisable to prevent bullying and unwanted sexual harassment.

The Rabbit Welfare Association and the Royal Society for the Prevention of Cruelty to Animals (RSPCA) advise keeping rabbits in pairs. Mullan and Main (2006) found that 56% of rabbits in their survey were kept with another rabbit.

It is not advised to keep guinea pigs with rabbits. This is probably more important for the guinea pig than the rabbit as they are often bullied and may form the focus of unwanted sexual attention particularly if housed with a male entire rabbit. In addition, rabbits commonly carry bacteria such as *Bordetella bronchiseptica* in their upper airways, and this may cause pneumonia in guinea pigs.

### 3.1.7 Checking the rabbit for problems

It is important that the rabbit is regularly checked for problems. Although this may seem obvious, many pet rabbits are kept and looked

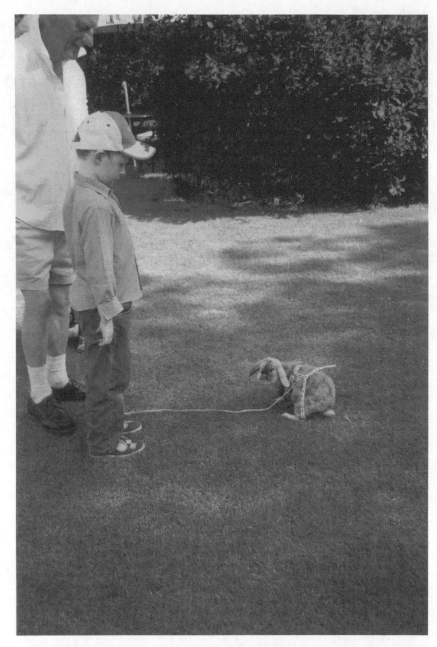

**Figure 3.3** The dangers of not securing the rabbit harness correctly can lead to escape and possible harm to the rabbit.

**Table 3.1** Commonly encountered problems of domestic rabbits

| Problem | Description |
| --- | --- |
| Dental disease | May be obvious misalignment or overgrowth of incisors. Problems with cheek teeth are more difficult to see; however, the rabbits may go off their food or develop abscesses, faecal matting of the rear or start pulling fur out over the body |
| Ear mites | Crusting of the ears and build-up of debris in the ear canals *Cheyletiella cuniculi* mites – dandruff and loss of fur seen initially dorsally, but may spread over the whole body. A reduction in grooming, such as may occur with dental disease, may act as the trigger for a *Cheyletiella* mite population explosion and clinical signs of infestation |
| Faecal matting | Collection of faeces around the anus and tail often associated with spinal problems, dental disease or digestive tract disturbances |
| Fly strike | Laying of eggs and production of maggots in soiled fur around the anus |
| Snuffles | Nasal discharge, wetness around the nose and mouth Abscess formation – swelling and pain often found around the head and associated with dental disease |
| Sore hocks | Redness, thickening, weeping and/or infection of the skin above the foot of the hind feet as the rabbit adopts a plantigrade stance and the hocks become weight bearing |

after by children, and therefore a list of the most common problems may prove helpful for them.

The most common problems encountered can be seen in Table 3.1.

### 3.1.8 Prevention of sunburn

White rabbits can suffer from the same skin problems as white cats and dogs. If they spend lots of time outside in bright sunlight, then the ears, which are poorly furred, can be affected by sunburn (see Fig. 3.4) which can eventually lead to malignant cancer (generally squamous cell carcinoma) as is seen in white furred cats and dogs. Applying sun block to the ears and reducing access to sunlight during the summer months can be helpful.

### 3.1.9 Vaccination

The two diseases for which vaccination is currently commercially available in the UK are myxomatosis and viral haemorrhagic disease. These conditions are discussed in more detail in the section on medical

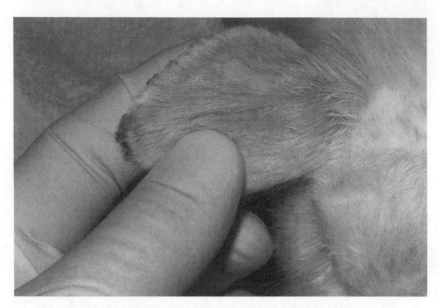

**Figure 3.4** Crusting of the ear margins in a white-furred rabbit indicative of early pre-cancerous changes associated with sunburn.

nursing (see Chapter 9). However, the main points that owners need to be aware of are as follows.

## Myxomatosis

This condition is caused by the myxoma virus carried principally by the rabbit flea, *S. cuniculi*. The virus acts systemically. Externally it affects the eyes, skin and external genitalia, causing swelling of the eyelids, base of the ears (eventually extending to the whole face) and the external genitalia (see Figs 3.5 and 3.6). A creamy oculonasal discharge is also commonly observed. The rabbit is pyrexic, often running a fever of 41–42°C and also anorexic. The condition is very difficult to manage and there is no known cure. In most cases the infection will be fatal.

The condition is found intermittently in wild rabbits, and therefore if there is any chance that the pet rabbit can come in contact with a wild rabbit or with cats or other animals that may be carrying rabbit fleas then they should be vaccinated. Vaccination can take place from 6 weeks of age and should be repeated every 6–12 months depending on veterinary advice.

It is still possible for rabbits that have been vaccinated to be affected by the condition, but in these cases the clinical signs are much less severe and supportive therapy is usually successful. In most cases they develop

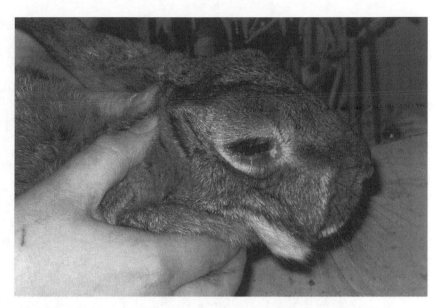

**Figure 3.5**  Myxomatosis lesions in a wild rabbit. Note the swelling around the eyes and base of the ears and common oculonasal milky discharge.

the cutaneous form of the disease with raised myxoma lesions appearing usually over the head, particularly around the nose.

### Viral haemorrhagic disease

Viral haemorrhagic disease is caused by a calicivirus and is transmitted from rabbit to rabbit or via fomites, the virus being able to survive in the environment for weeks rather than days. The disease can cause sudden death, convulsions, epistaxis, hepatitis, jaundice and respiratory distress.

As for myxomatosis, no treatment is curative and the condition is generally fatal. Vaccination is available to rabbits 10–12 weeks old and should be repeated every 6–12 months. In the case of an outbreak where younger rabbits are present, they may be vaccinated at less than 10 weeks of age, but the vaccine should be repeated after 1 month.

## 3.2 House rabbits

You will be well aware of the increase in popularity of house rabbits over the past few years. As the name suggests house rabbits spend most

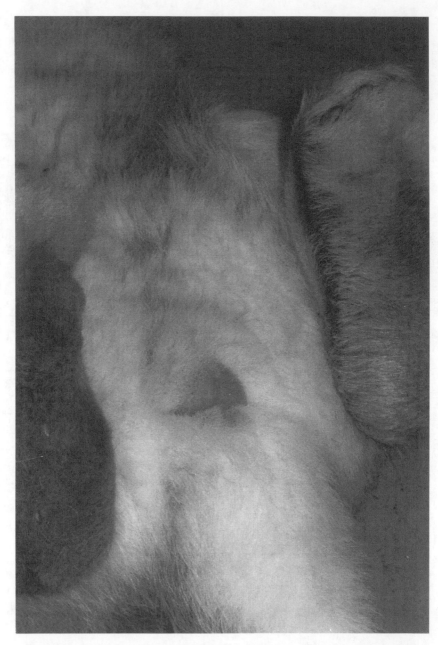

**Figure 3.6**  Myxomatosis lesions in a wild rabbit. Note the anogenital swelling.

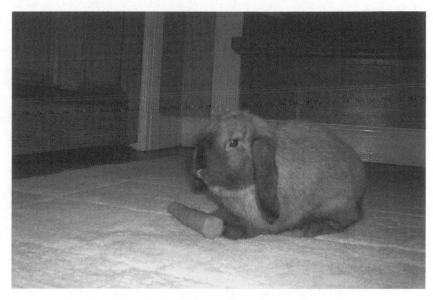

**Figure 3.7** A typical house rabbit. Courtesy of Adam Bisset.

of their time in the house with their owner and possibly other pets (see Fig. 3.7). However, they also need to have access to the outside – either an enclosed escape proof garden, or a run area.

Within the house the rabbit needs to have a bed area that they regard as their safe area. Remember that the rabbit is a prey species and if frightened the rabbit needs a bolt-hole. The cage can be a box or similar structure lined with straw/hay or alternatively a commercial outdoor hutch may be used. If the rabbit is allowed access to more than one room in the house then it may be helpful to provide more than one such bolt-hole. Large cardboard tubes that the rabbit can hide in are also helpful.

The two main areas that owners will require information about are house training and preventing chewing of various structures within the house.

### 3.2.1 House training

Rabbits are generally clean animals and will select one specific area to use as a toilet, usually in a corner of a room or along a wall. Providing them with a litter tray containing litter material in a quiet secluded area of the room may be enough to litter train the rabbit. Placing food bowls in other corners of the room can prevent the rabbit from using these areas.

During early litter training, confining the rabbit to its hutch/pen area can help in allowing it associate its tray with urination/defaecation. As with most young animals, rabbits will tend to urinate/defaecate after feeding. Therefore, confining the rabbit to its pen area with litter tray at feeding time will usually encourage the rabbit to use this as the toilet area.

Material used for litter can include straw, paper, or cat litter. The only material that should be avoided are clay-based cat litters because if eaten then this can cause an impaction.

Entire male rabbits will mark their territory with urine, and therefore it may be best to neuter if considering keeping them as a house rabbit.

### 3.2.2 Chewing

Rabbits will chew their surroundings and this is something that owners need to be prepared for. Cables need to be covered, items that the owner does not wish to be chewed should be kept out of reach, and any house plants thought or known to be poisonous to rabbits should be removed. Providing toys and material for the rabbit to chew may help, but it is likely that the rabbit will chew something in their surroundings at some point.

Distracting the rabbit by thumping on the floor with the hand or foot can work with some rabbits as this mimics the rabbit warning signal. Alternatively using a water pistol to fire a stream of water at the rabbit if caught in the act can be effective.

Some household items are potentially very dangerous to rabbits, a good example would be electric cabling. In many cases it may not be possible to prevent rabbits from chewing these; therefore, rooms where cabling cannot be elevated off the floor or encased in chew-proof material should probably be out of bounds for the house rabbit.

### 3.2.3 Toys

Items that are non-toxic and unlikely to cause a gut obstruction are suitable toys for rabbits. Examples include cardboard tubes such as the inner toilet roll tubes, writing paper scrunched into balls, pieces of vegetable such as carrot or turnip that may be rolled around the floor.

Some rabbits, particularly single house rabbits, can be provided with a stuffed toy as a 'cage mate' to cuddle up to. Care should be taken to inspect the toy regularly to ensure it is not being eaten, and any external features that are easily dislodged should be removed from the toy before giving it to the rabbit. Alternatively, an old dishtowel wrapped around scrunched-up writing paper can make a relatively innocuous toy.

## 3.3 Grooming

Self-grooming is a normal aspect of rabbit behaviour as for the majority of animals. However, this may not occur for a number of reasons, e.g. neurological problems/spinal problems that may result in poor proprioception, or dental problems that make grooming painful. As you have seen already there are great differences in the physical appearance of different rabbit breeds. Short-coated breeds are usually able to groom themselves. Long-haired breeds such as the Angora however will need some form of daily grooming. Also, any rabbits with dental disease or spinal problems such as spondylosis or rabbits that are overweight will have problems grooming themselves. If grooming is carried out when the rabbits are young then it can provide a chance for the owner to check the rabbit over regularly for any problems.

Bathing is not something that is routinely carried out in rabbits. Although it is not impossible to bathe a rabbit, most rabbits do not appreciate being placed in a bowl of water and will try to escape. Unless the rabbit has been in a particularly muddy run, or has faecal matting, bathing is not required. Fine long-haired breeds such as the Angora should not be bathed if at all possible as the fur mats very easily.

## 3.4 Rabbits in the practice

Caring for a rabbit within the practice follows the same principles as those described already for owners at home (see Fig. 3.8).

The cage should be situated in an area away from cats and dogs and noise in order to minimise stress levels. The cage should be small enough so that the nurse can reach the rabbit, but also large enough to allow the rabbit to move around. Water should be provided in a container similar to that used at home – either a water bottle situated at a suitable height for the rabbit or in a bowl.

Bedding should be provided to prevent the formation of hock sores. Straw is not advisable and newspaper or incontinence pads are preferable, although rabbits are likely to chew any form of bedding that is provided. House rabbits can also be provided with a litter tray using a substrate that the rabbit is used to.

**Table 3.2** Examples of disinfectants used in rabbit veterinary practice

| Trade name | Active ingredient | Indications | Notes |
|---|---|---|---|
| Ammonia | 10% ammonia | Killing coccidial oocysts (Pakes and Gerrity, 1994) | Hazardous substance. Use with extreme caution |
| Ark-Klens® (Vetark Professional) | Benzalkonium chloride | Bacterial and fungal infections | |
| F10® (Health and Hygiene (Pty) Ltd) | Quarternary ammonium compounds + biguanides + tetrasodium EDTA + nonylphenol oxide condensate | Bacterial, viral and fungal infections | |
| Tamodine-E® (Vetark Professional) | Povidone-iodine | Bacterial, viral and fungal infections | |
| TriGene® (MediChem International) | Halogenated tertiary amine | Bacterial, viral and fungal infections | |
| Virkon® (DuPont Animal Health Solutions) | Oxidising agent | Bacterial, viral and fungal infections | Potentially irritant to the skin |

Please note that this table is not intended to be an exhaustive list of available disinfectants.

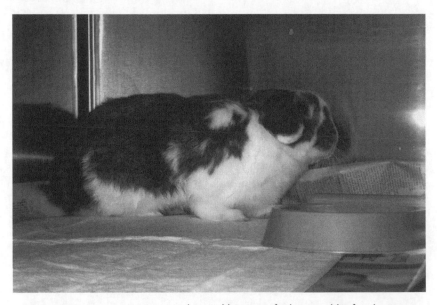

**Figure 3.8** Common veterinary hospital housing of a house rabbit for short-term procedures.

One area that may be significantly different is the presence of transmissible disease which is likely to be higher in the veterinary practice than the home. In these cases cages and contents such as food bowls need to be regularly disinfected. For steel cages or cages with an impervious surface, disinfectants that are effective against principally bacteria, parasites and viruses such as *Pasteurella* spp., coccidia and viral haemorrhagic disease, respectively, are advisable as these are common rabbit pathogens. A list of commonly used disinfectants is given in Table 3.2.

# References

Home Office (2003) *Code of Practice for the Housing and Care of Animals Used in Scientific Procedure*, The Stationery Office, London.

DEFRA (2008) *Codes of Recommendations for the Welfare of Livestock Rabbits*. This can be accessed via the DEFRA website at http://www.defra.gov.uk/animalh/welfare/farmed/othersps/rabbits/pb0080/rabcode.htm (accessed on 23/11/08).

Meredith, A. and Crossley, D.A. (2002) Rabbits. In: *Manual of Exotic Pets*, 4th edn (eds, Meredith, A. and Redrobe, S.P.), BSAVA, Quedgeley, Gloucestershire, pp. 76–92.

Mullan, S.M. and Main, D.C.J. (2006) Survey of the husbandry, health and welfare of 102 pet rabbits. *Veterinary Record* 159:103–109.

Pakes, S.P. and Gerrity, L.W. (1994) Protozoal diseases. In: *The Biology of the Laboratory Rabbit*, 2nd edn (eds, Manning, P.J., Ringler, D.H. and Newcomer, C.E.) San Diego, London.

RSPCA (2003) Rabbits. In: *Animal Care Leaflet*, RSPCA Publications, Horsham.

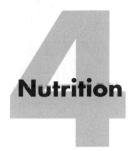

# Nutrition 4

## 4.1 General nutritional requirements

### 4.1.1 Water

Water quality is important as many rabbits will dunk food in their water supply, or if the water feeders are poorly situated at low levels in bowls rather than sip feeders, some rabbits may actually defaecate in the water bowls. This can lead to massive bacterial population explosions and potentially lead to gastroenteritis. Another factor to consider in water quality is the administration of mineral/vitamin supplements as these will allow rapid bacterial growth in the enriched water.

The amount of water consumed by individual rabbits will obviously depend on the diets being offered and the species considered. On dry pellet-based diets water consumption will be much higher than for diets where consumption of large amounts of fresh vegetables and fresh grass occurs. An average 2-kg rabbit may consume 200 mL or more water in a day if fed a completely dry diet.

### 4.1.2 Maintenance energy requirements

Every species has a level of energy consumption per day needed to satisfy basic maintenance requirements that is energy used purely to maintain current status under minimal activity and hence is frequently the lowest energy requirement during that mammal's life. In relation to other species, a formula has been derived as maintenance energy requirements (MER) are dependent on the basal metabolic rate (the energy requirement when at complete rest). The MER is calculated as follows:

$$MER = constant\,(k) \times (body\ weight)^{0.75}$$

The constant, $k$, varies with family groups, and has been estimated at 100 for adult rabbits, going up to 200 for growth and 300 for lactation (Carpenter and Kolmstetter, 2000).

Energy requirements give a guide to what a rabbit must consume per day in order to continue to maintain good health and body weight. Hence, if the foods offered are so low in kilojoules/calorie that the rabbit has to eat more of it than will fit into its digestive system in 24 hours, the rabbit will rapidly lose condition.

An example is that of high water vegetable foods such as lettuce have a low energy density of 3 kcal/g weight dry matter (0.18 kcal/g real/wet weight). In this case lettuce on its own is unlikely to meet the requirements of a high energy-demanding lactating doe which has a requirement of 200–300 kcal (837–1255 kJ) ME/kg body weight daily (Carpenter and Kolmstetter, 2000).

Conversely, rabbits are concentrate selectors and so will choose the higher fat foods present in their environment in preference to low fat ones. Therefore, if offered these foods *ad libitum* the propensity to become obese is high.

## 4.1.3 Protein and amino acid requirements

The ten essential amino acids required by other mammals are also needed by the rabbits, and the concept of biological value of a protein is just as applicable. In addition, it is known that diets low in the amino acids, methionine or arginine, an extra supplement of the amino acid glycine is required.

For rabbits, levels of protein content in the diet have been shown to vary from 15 to 18% as dry matter (Hillyer *et al.*, 1997). A study looking at differing levels of protein from 16 to 24% fed to gravid does showed that there was no significant difference in gestation length, litter size and the number of kittens dead at birth (Iyeghe-Erakpotobor *et al.*, 2005). However, the same study showed that individual kitten weight at birth increased with protein levels and those does fed at 24% crude protein produced kittens that had a higher growth rate than those fed at 18 or

20%. In rabbits the majority of the proteins are from plant sources such as clover, alfalfa hay and good quality grass hays.

### 4.1.4 Fats and essential fatty acids

Fats provide high concentrations of energy but also supply the rabbit with essential fatty acids required for cellular integrity and as the building blocks for internal chemicals such as prostaglandins which play a part in reproduction and inflammation.

Fats also provide a carrier mechanism for the absorption of fat-soluble vitamins such as vitamin A, D, E and K.

The primary essential fatty acid for rabbits is linoleic acid as it is for larger mammals, with the absolute dietary requirement of this fatty acid being 1% of the diet. If the diet becomes deficient in this essential fatty acid, a rapid decline in cellular integrity occurs which is manifested clinically by the skin becoming flaky and dry and prone to recurrent infections, and also to fluid loss through the skin which in turn leads to polydipsia. Rabbits require no additional dietary fat other than the 2–5% provided in their vegetable-based diet.

Another essential fatty acid which is thought to be important is alpha-linolenic acid which is necessary for some prostaglandin/eicosanoid production.

In rabbits, because of their much lower requirement for fat, excess plant fats can cause severe hepatic lipidosis and atherosclerosis in the aorta. Sources of sunflower and other high oil-based seeds are often the culprits.

### 4.1.5 Carbohydrates

In rabbits most of the carbohydrates required are in the form of fibre. It is important for many reasons. Fibre provides a source of abrasive food, as most of the fibre providing foods, such as grasses, contain silicates, all of which wear down the teeth. This is important as rabbits have continually erupting teeth, which will grow even if there is no wearing of the teeth occurring, and needs to be kept in check.

Secondly, the fibre is essential to stimulate gut motility, as rabbits are hindgut fermenters and rely on the microflora of the hindgut to digest food by breaking down the cellulose. Without sufficient fibre, rabbits can experience a digestive disturbance, with intermittent constipation, diarrhoea and colic. Fibre becomes converted by the intestinal microflora into volatile fatty acids, which decrease the pH of the caecum and large bowel, so preventing bacterial overgrowth and minimising enteritis problems. The volatile fatty acids are absorbed into the bloodstream and converted by the liver into glucose that the body can use for energy.

Rabbits have a requirement for 12–16% crude fibre (Carpenter and Kolmstetter, 2000). It is recommended therefore that rabbits are fed fresh grass, good quality hay, or dried grass/dried grass pellets as 30–50% of their diet as a minimum. The sole feeding of pelleted/dry mix foods currently available can lead to a major fibre shortage, which leads to lack of dental wear and gastrointestinal upsets and promotes obesity.

## 4.1.6 Fat-soluble vitamins

### Vitamin A

In rabbits the diet frequently contains only the vitamin A precursors as carotenoid plant pigments, with beta-carotene being the most important.

Hypovitaminosis A is an uncommonly seen rabbit disease. This is because green vegetables are good providers of the beta-carotenes. Hypovitaminosis A in rabbits can cause infertility, foetal resorptions, abortions, stillbirths and neurological defects such as hydrocephalus. Recommendations for diets include 7000 IU/kg for rabbits (Carpenter and Kolmstetter, 2000). The low levels may be met by as little as 200 g of carrot per day for a 2-kg rabbit, but would require 70 kg of oats to provide the same levels.

Vitamin A, because it is fat soluble, can be stored in the body, primarily in the liver.

Hypervitaminosis A rarely occurs naturally but may be induced by overdosing with vitamin A injections at 1000 times or more the daily recommended doses. If this occurs acute toxicity develops with mucus membrane and skin sloughing, liver damage and frequently death within 24–48 hours.

### Vitamin D

This vitamin is primarily concerned with calcium metabolism in the body.

Cholecalciferol is manufactured in the rabbit's skin, a process enhanced by ultraviolet light, hence indoor rabbits produce much less of this compound which can lead to deficiencies. This compound must then be activated first in the liver and kidneys before it is functional in calcium metabolism. Once formed into its active metabolite, it functions in concert with parathyroid hormone (PTH) to increase reabsorption of calcium at the expense of phosphorus from the kidneys and to mobilise calcium from the bones all of these functions increasing the blood calcium levels. It does not however have any effect on calcium absorption from the gut as in rabbits this rate is permanently 'set' at a maximum level which can lead to problems with calcium over-supplementation such as urolithiasis and soft tissue mineralisation.

Hypovitaminosis D3 therefore as mentioned causes problems with calcium metabolism and leads to rickets. This is exacerbated by low calcium-containing diets, a typical sufferer being an indoor kept rabbit fed an inappropriate seed/cereal-based diet. This leads to well-muscled heavy rabbits, but poorly mineralised bones and flaring of the epiphyseal plates at the ends of the long bones, with concomitant bowing of the limbs, especially the tibiotarsal bones. Recommended minimum levels are 3.5–9 IU/g of feed for rabbits (Wallach and Hoff, 1982).

Hypervitaminosis D3 occurs due to over-supplementation with D3 and calcium, and leads to calcification of soft tissues such as the arteries medial walls and the kidneys, creating hypertension and organ failure.

Recommended maximum levels are 2000 IU/kg dry matter for most small mammals (Wallach and Hoff, 1982).

### Vitamin E

This compound is found in several active forms in plants, the most active being alpha-tocopherol. It is used as an antioxidant and in immune system function in the body.

Hypovitaminosis E in rabbits is occasionally seen with hindlimb paresis and white muscle degeneration. Hypovitaminosis E may occur due to a reduction in fat metabolism or absorption as can occur in small intestinal/pancreatic/biliary diseases, or due to a lack of green plant material, the chief source of the compound, in the diet. Recommended levels for rabbits are 40 mg/kg dry matter of food offered (National Research Council, 1978). Hypervitaminosis E is extremely rare.

### Vitamin K

Because of the production of vitamin K by bacteria, it is very difficult to get its true deficiency, although absorption will again be reduced when fat digestion/absorption is reduced as in, for example, biliary or pancreatic disease.

The consumption of warfarin or other coumerol-containing rodenticides may lead to a relative deficiency in rabbits. Feeding large amounts of sweet clovers that contain coumerol derivatives can also cause a relative deficiency. Disease caused is due to increased internal and external haemorrhage, but vitamin K has also some function in calcium/phosphorous metabolism in the bones and this may also be affected.

## 4.1.7 Water-soluble vitamins

### Vitamin B1 (thiamine)

Hypovitaminosis B1 is uncommon in rabbits as it is found widely in green vegetable matter. Recommended minimum level for most small mammals lies around 6–7 mg/kg of diet dry matter (Wallach and Hoff, 1982).

### Vitamin B2 (riboflavin)

Hypovitaminosis B2 is very rare and produces growth retardation and roughened coat, alopecia and excess scurf and cataract formation.

### Niacin

Rabbits fed a high proportion of one type of seed, such as sweetcorn, can become deficient with blackening of the tongue (known as pellagra) and oral mucosa, retarded growth, poor coat quality and scaly dermatitis.

### Biotin

Deficiencies produce exfoliative dermatitis, toes may become gangrenous and slough off and ataxia may be observed. Again deficiencies are rare. Recommended minimum requirements are 0.12–0.34 ppm food as dry matter for small mammals (Wallach and Hoff, 1982).

### Folic acid

Deficiencies occur mainly due to the existence of inhibitors to folic acid in some foods such as cabbage and other brassicas, oranges, beans and peas, and the use of trimethoprim sulphonamide drugs also reduces gut bacterial folic acid production. This can lead to a number of obvious problems such as failure in reproductive tract maturation, macrocytic anaemia due to failure of red blood cell maturation and immune system cellular dysfunction.

### Choline

Because of interactions, the need for choline is dependant on levels of folic acid and vitamin B12, which may cause deficiencies if they themselves are deficient as does a diet high in fats. Deficiencies cause retarded growth, disrupted fat metabolism, and fatty liver damage. Recommended minimum requirements are 880–1540 mg/kg food as dry matter for small mammals.

### Vitamin C

There is no direct need for this vitamin in rabbits as vitamin C may be produced from glucose in the liver. However during disease processes, particularly those which affect the liver function, it may be beneficial to the recovery process to provide a dietary source of vitamin C. It is required for the formation of elastic fibres and connective tissues and is an excellent antioxidant similar to vitamin E. Deficiencies lead to 'scurvy' where there is poor wound healing, increased bleeding due to capillary wall fragility, gingivitis and bone alterations such as swelling of the long bones close to joints (the epiphyseal plates), which become very painful. In addition, crusting occurs at mucocutaneous junctions such as the eyes, mouth and nose as well as loosening of the teeth due to periodontal ligament weakening.

Vitamin C does actually also help in the absorption from the gut in some minerals such as iron.

## 4.1.8 Macrominerals

### Calcium

Calcium has a wide range of bodily functions, the two most obvious being its role in the formation of the skeleton/mineralisation of bone matrix and its requirement for muscular contractions. The active form of calcium in the body is the ionic double-charged molecule $Ca^{2+}$. Low levels of this form, even though the overall body reserves of calcium are normal, leads to hyperexcitability, fitting and death.

Calcium levels in the body are controlled by vitamin D3, PTH and calcitonin. Vitamin D3 promotes calcium retention in the kidneys and affects mobilisation of calcium from bones and absorption from the gut. Calcitonin decreases blood calcium levels by promoting excretion of calcium from the kidneys and by deposition into the bones. PTH increases blood calcium levels by promoting calcium resorption from the bones and by increasing the rate of conversion of vitamin D2 (25-hydroxycholecalciferol) to vitamin D3 (1,25-dihydroxycholecalciferol) in the kidneys.

The ratio of calcium to phosphorus is also important. As one increases, the other decreases and vice versa. Therefore a ratio of 2:1 calcium to phosphorus is desirable in most situations. Excessive calcium in the diet (>1%) reduces the use of proteins, fats, phosphorus, manganese, zinc, iron and iodine, and in rabbits leads to excess calcium excretion into the urine with the formation of calcium carbonate crystals and urolithiasis. This is exacerbated by the rabbit's unique method of calcium control in that there is no ability to down-regulate calcium absorption from the gut in the rabbit as occurs in other species. Instead all available calcium is absorbed from the diet, and any excess must then be excreted through the kidneys. In addition as rabbits are herbivorous, their urine pH is alkaline, and calcium carbonate (limestone) is less soluble in alkaline environments and so precipitates readily in the urine, forming crystals. Levels of calcium >4% dry matter for rabbits will lead to soft tissue mineralisation such as the aorta and kidneys.

A low dietary calcium level in young growing rabbits has been linked with dental disease due to the creation of 'metabolic bone disease' and loss of alveolar bone around the apex of the teeth (Harcourt-Brown, 1996). This leads to a lack of dental support, loosening of the teeth, progression of the apex of the teeth through the periosteum of the jawbones and altered wear of the teeth. Increased PTH levels are suggestive of metabolic bone disease in the rabbit (Harcourt-Brown and Baker, 2001).

## Phosphorus

Phosphorus is, as calcium, utilised in bone formation, but also cell structure and energy storage. It is widespread in plants and animal tissues, but the former may be bound up in unavailable forms as phytates. Levels of phosphorus are controlled in the body as for calcium, the two being in equal and opposite equilibrium with each other. Therefore, if dietary levels exceed calcium levels appreciably (a maximum of twice the calcium levels on average), the parathyroid glands become stimulated to produce more PTH and nutritional secondary hyperparathyroidism occurs which leads to progressive bone demineralisation and renal damage due to high circulating levels of PTH. High dietary phosphorus also reduces the amount of calcium which can be absorbed from the gut as it complexes with the calcium present there. Green vegetables, good quality hay or supplementation with calcium powders may therefore be necessary.

### Potassium

As with larger mammals, this is the major intracellular positive ion. Rarely is there a dietary deficiency, but severe stress can cause hypokalaemia due to increased kidney excretion of potassium as a result of elevated plasma proteins, as can persistent diarrhoea, which can lead to cardiac dysrhythmias, muscle spasticity and neurological dysfunction. Other symptoms present as stunted growth, ascites, abnormally short hair and reduced appetite. It is present in high amounts in certain fruits such as bananas and is controlled in the body in equilibrium with sodium under the influence of the adrenal hormone aldosterone which promotes sodium retention and potassium excretion.

### Sodium

This is the main extracellular positive ion and regulates the body's acid base balance and osmotic potential. In conjunction with potassium, it is responsible for nerve signals/impulses. Rarely does a true dietary deficiency occur, but hyponatraemia may occur due to chronic diarrhoea or renal disease. This disrupts the osmotic potential gradient in the kidneys and water is lost leading to further dehydration. Excessive levels of sodium in the diet (>10 times recommended) lead to poor coat, polyuria, hypertension, oedema and death.

### Chlorine

This is the major extracellular negative ion and responsible for maintaining acid-base balances in conjunction with sodium and potassium.

Deficiencies are rare, but if they do occur, retarded growth and kidney disease are commonly seen.

## 4.1.9 Trace elements/microminerals

### *Iodine*

Iodine's sole function is in thyroid hormone synthesis, which affects metabolic rate. Deficiencies cause goitre, and have knock-on effects on reduced growth stunting, stillbirths and neurological problems. It is a relatively uncommon finding in rabbits but may be seen when they are fed large volumes of goitrogenic (iodine-inhibiting) plants such as cabbage, kale and Brussel sprouts.

### *Iron*

This is essential as with other mammals for the formation of the oxygen, carrying part of the haemoglobin molecule. Absorption from the gut is normally relatively poor, as the body is very good at recycling its iron levels. Deficiencies are rare.

### *Manganese*

Deficiencies have been reported as causing poor bone growth with limb shortening as a consequence. Recommended daily requirements are from 40 to 120.7 ppm (Wallach and Hoff, 1982).

### *Selenium*

The main role of selenium is as part of the antioxidant enzyme glutathione peroxidase which vitamin E is also involved in. Its functions are therefore similar to vitamin E in that it helps neutralise peroxidases from attacking polyunsaturated fats in cell membranes; a general deficiency in both selenium and vitamin E will lead to liver necrosis, steatitis and muscular dystrophy. Selenium content of plants is dependant on where they were grown and the levels of selenium in the soil. Recommended minimum requirements are still not clearly defined for small mammals in general.

*Zinc*

This is a vital trace element for wound healing and tissue formation, forming part of a number of enzymes. Deficiencies can occur in young rapidly growing rabbits fed on plant material high in phytates such as cabbage, wheat bran and beans. In addition, high dietary calcium decreases the zinc uptake. Deficiencies produce retarded growth and poor skin quality with increased scurf and hyperirritability. Minimum recommended requirements are 20–122 ppm for small mammals (Wallach and Hoff, 1982).

## 4.2 Requirements for young and lactating rabbits

Neonatal rabbits nurse for only 3–5 minutes at a time once or twice in a 24-hour period and are totally dependant on their mother's milk up to day 21 post-parturition (Okerman, 1994). At this time they should be weighed, as solid foods offered will be increasingly consumed and weight losses may be seen. The doe may be offered increasingly more pelleted dry foods, as her energy demands rise to 3.5 times maintenance by peak lactation. Ad lib dry food is therefore often advocated for the doe at this stage. It should be noted though that levels of food for the doe should not start to be dramatically increased until 5–7 days after parturition as early overfeeding can lead to mastitis due to too much milk production which outstrips the kits' appetite to empty the mammary glands at each sitting.

Rabbit kittens are difficult to rear artificially. Many females will not foster a strange doe's kittens, but does kept together, and lactating at the same time will often allow the suckling of the other's young. This is the best scenario if another known lactating doe is available. If not, as is often the case, hand rearing may be attempted. A rearing formula has been derived (Okerman, 1994) comprising 25 mL of whole cows' milk to 75 mL of condensed milk and 6 g of lyophilised skimmed milk powder. A vitamin supplement may be added to this. The kitten is fed twice a day only, from 2 to 10 mL depending on the age. This should continue until the kitten is 2 weeks old when more and more good quality hay and pellets should be introduced, aiming to wean the kitten at 3 weeks. The anogenital area should be stimulated with a piece of damp cotton wool after every feed to stimulate urination and defaecation for the first 2 weeks.

Growing kits require higher levels of vitamin D3 and calcium than their adult counterparts. To ensure that this is received, a balanced diet should be offered – a combination of a pelleted food, good quality grass hay and some greens is advised. The pelleted foods should be carefully chosen. Many are balanced nutritionally, but only if the rabbit consumes all parts equally. If given pellets ad lib, as rabbits are concentrate selectors (that is they will preferentially pick out those foods containing the highest calories in their environment and eat them first), they will eat all of the fatty, carbohydrate foods first, and if provided in quantity, they will not get around to eating the high fibre, calcium-containing grass pellets. Hence, using a homogenous pelleted diet where all of the pellets are exactly the same, or feeding enough in 24 hours so that the bowl is completely emptied before offering more is advised. Access to unfiltered natural sunlight is also advised, even if for only 15–20 minutes per day, to ensure sufficient vitamin D3 synthesis. Lactating does will also have higher calcium requirements, and so their consumption of pelleted diet and grass products (both high in calcium) will increase.

## 4.3 Requirements for debilitated rabbits

In general, requirements for debilitated species will vary from 1.5 to 3 times maintenance levels, with the lower levels being for mildly injured / infected animals and the upper levels for burns victims, serious organ damage or septicaemic cases.

The use of fluid therapy as additional support is essential, particularly for the herbivorous mammals owing to their increased maintenance requirements over cats and dogs (average 80–100 mL/kg/day). Also, the gut contents are voluminous in herbivores and need to be kept fluid. For further details see chapter 9 on small mammal therapeutics.

The debilitated rabbit may be supported with nasogastric or oral syringing of vegetable-based baby foods (lactose-free varieties), or more ideally with a gruel composed of ground dry rabbit pellets and water as the latter has a better fibre level for gut stimulation. More recently specific liquid feed formulas have been derived for rabbits and other small herbivores by commercial manufacturer, see Chapter 10. Amounts suggested at any one sitting vary from 3 to 15 mL four to six times daily. A nasogastric tube (more correctly a naso-oesophageal tube as the tubing must not allow reflux of acidic stomach contents into the oesophagus) is placed after first spraying the nose with lignocaine spray and inserting the 3–4 French tube which has been pre-measured from the extended nose to the seventh rib or caudal end of the sternum. Sterile water should be flushed through the tube before and after feeding to ensure it is correctly placed and does not become blocked. The tube may then be glued, taped or sutured to the dorsal aspect of the head and a bung inserted when not in use. It may be necessary to put an Elizabethan collar on the rabbit to prevent removal.

The use of cisapride (0.5 mg/kg orally every 8–24 hours; Smith and Bergmann, 1997) or metoclopramide (0.2–0.5 mg/kg orally every 6–8 hours) with ranitidine (2–5 mg/kg orally every 12 hours) is to be advocated in rabbits to stimulate large bowel activity and encourage a return to appetite.

Older rabbits often do better on lower protein (levels of 14%) and higher fibre (18%) diets as these reduce the risk of obesity and kidney and liver damage.

### 4.3.1 Probiotics

The use of oral probiotics is controversial as a study has shown that *Enterococcus faecalis* and *Enterococcus faecium* are the predominant enterococcal species in the gut of rabbits (Linaje *et al.*, 2004) although the predominant bacteria of the commercial probiotic are *Lactobacillus* spp. However, Hollister *et al.* (1989 and 1990) have shown that probiotics were effective in reducing the incidence of enteritis as well as increasing weight gain in recently weaned kittens. Probiotics are best added to the drinking water but may be added to the syringed food to ensure consumption. No ill effects have been reported with their use and so the worst-case scenario seems that they will do no harm as well as no good. In general, this author has found that commercial probiotics available are preferable to no probiotic or caecotroph use at all and aid return to normal gut function in debilitated rabbits.

The use of gavaging or stomach tubing a sick rabbit with the caecotrophs of a healthy rabbit is also beneficial and likely to aid recolonisation of the gut with normal bacteria and protozoa. It is often easier to blend the caecotrophs with a pureed vegetable baby food to encourage acceptance.

## References

Carpenter, J.W. and Kolmstetter, C.M. (2000) Feeding small exotic mammals. In: *Hills Nutrition*, Mark Mervis Institute, Marceline, Missouri, pp. 943–960.

Harcourt-Brown, F.M. (1996) Calcium deficiency, diet and dental disease in pet rabbits. *Veterinary Record* 139:567–571.

Harcourt-Brown, F.M. and Baker, S.J. (2001) Parathyroid hormone, haematological and biochemical parameters in relation to dental disease and husbandry in pet rabbits. *Journal of Small Animal Practice* 42:130–136.

Hillyer, E.V., Quesenberry, K.E. and Donnelly, T.M (1997) Biology, husbandry and clinical techniques. In: *Ferrets, Rabbits and Rodents: Clinical Medicine and Surgery* (eds, Hillyer, E.V. and Quesenberry, K.E.), WB Saunders, Philadelphia, pp. 243–259.

Hollister, A.G., Cheeke, P.R., Robinson, K.L. and Patton, N.M. (1989) Effects of water-administered probiotics and acidifiers on growth, feed conversion and enteritis mortality of weanling rabbits. *Journal of Applied Rabbit Research* 12:143–147.

Hollister, A.G., Cheeke, P.R., Robinson, K.L. and Patton, N.M. (1990) Effects of dietary probiotics and acidifiers on performance of weanling rabbits. *Journal of Applied Rabbit Research* 13:6–9.

Iyeghe-Erakpotobor, G.T., Olorunju, A.S. and Oyedipe, E.O. (2005) Effect of protein level and flushing method on the reproductive performance of rabbits. *Animal Science Journal* 76:209–215.

Linaje, R., Coloma, M.D., Pérez-Martinez, G. and Zuniga, M. (2004) Characterisation of faecal enterococci from rabbits for the selection of probiotic strains. *Journal of Applied Microbiology* 96:761–771.

National Research Council (1978) *Nutrient Requirements of Laboratory Animals*, National Academy Press, Washington, DC.

Okerman, L. (1994) Breeding problems. In: *Diseases of Domestic Rabbits*, 2nd edn, Blackwell Scientific Publications, Oxford, pp. 113–120.

Smith, D.A. and Bergmann, P.M. (1997) Formulary. In: *Ferrets, Rabbits and Rodents: Clinical Medicine and Surgery* (eds, Hillyer, E.V. and Quesenberry K.E.), WB Saunders, Philadelphia, pp. 392–403.

Wallach, J.D. and Hoff, G.L. (1982) Nutritional diseases of mammals. In: *Noninfectious Diseases of Wildlife* (eds, Hoff, G.L. and Davis, J.W.), Iowa State University Press, Ames, Iowa, pp. 133–135, 143–144.

# Further reading

Brooks, D.L. (2004) Nutrition and Gastrointestinal Physiology. In: *Ferrets, Rabbits and Rodents: Clinical Medicine and Surgery*, 2nd edn (eds, Quesenberry, K.E. and Carpenter, J.W.), Saunders, St. Louis, Missouri, pp. 155–160.

Harcourt-Brown, F. (2002) Diet and husbandry. In: Textbook of Rabbit Medicine, Butterworth Heineman, Edinburgh, pp. 19–51.

Kupersmith, D.S. (1998) A practical overview of small mammal nutrition. *Seminars in Avian and Exotic Pet Medicine* 7(3):141–147.

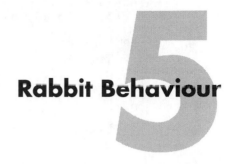

# Rabbit Behaviour

## 5.1 Normal behaviour

### 5.1.1 Introduction

Although pet rabbits have been bred for many years and look very different from their wild ancestor, when it comes to behaviour, pet rabbits still retain much of the behaviour found in wild rabbits.

The main fact that controls all rabbit behaviour is they are prey species. Therefore, fright and flight responses will control a lot of their responses. Giving the rabbits a protected environment where they are not placed under any stress and allowed to exhibit their natural behaviour will prevent the development of many behavioural problems that are presented in practice.

The main features of rabbit behaviour are listed in Box 5.1.

### 5.1.2 Socialisation and social interaction

Rabbits show some similarities to other species in that they should be socialised when young. The sensitive period has been shown to be 10–20 days (Kersten *et al.*, 1989). Rabbits introduced to humans and handling at this time will be much more responsive than rabbits that are not handled. Jezierski *et al.* (1993) have also demonstrated that handling rabbits at 3 months of age will affect the response to handling when these rabbits are adult. Therefore, when owners are buying a rabbit, it is important to find out how well the rabbit has been socialised or handled from a young

---

**Box 5.1   Features of natural rabbit behaviour**

- Prey species so respond in fright and flight manner
- Territorial
- Fixed periods of exercise and rest throughout the day
- Social animals that interact with other rabbits and other species
- Chewing is a normal behaviour
- Demonstrate fear by thumping or sometimes aggression
- Behaviour affected by sexual maturity and stage of reproductive cycle, e.g. bucks and does can become aggressive at sexual maturity; does may nest build and will often run around owner's legs, making grunting noises when in heat
- Spraying urine (neutering significantly reduces this but neutered rabbits may still spray urine)

---

age. Buying a rabbit that has never been handled can prove a challenge for the new owner. Where the rabbit is bought as a pet for a child, it can be distressing for all involved if the rabbit kicks and scratches every time that is it handled.

In the wild, rabbits are both social and territorial, living in social groups in large warrens. No matter how good the environment is, it is impossible to recreate this for domestic outdoor or house rabbits. As part of their territorial behaviour, rabbits will mark their territory. They do this by rubbing chin scent glands on their surroundings, urine spraying or placement of faecal pellets. Where rabbits are kept outside this behaviour will not cause any problems, but where rabbits are kept indoors this behaviour may need to be modified or controlled.

## 5.1.3 Feeding patterns

In the wild, rabbits tend to feed at dawn and dusk. This time will be spent grazing and travelling over a large area. Compare this with hutch rabbits that are presented with their food and can spend all of this time eating. It is hardly surprising that many pet rabbits can be overweight. Nutrition is discussed in Chapter 4, but it is important that owners realise that weight gain is a possibility and that rabbits are fed a variety of foods, some of low calorie such as hay, and that they are not fed large amounts of commercial pellets or rabbit mix.

House rabbits can be encouraged to forage for their food by hiding food in various areas throughout the rooms to which rabbits are allowed access. Again offering a variety of foods to the rabbit is important.

### 5.1.4 Activity and exercise

Rabbits require a lot of exercise and if given the opportunity can spend hours running or jumping around their environment. For hutch rabbits access to a run or enclosed garden is essential – although it is sadly not entirely true to say gone are the days when rabbits spent their entire life in a hutch at the bottom of the garden.

House rabbits will have access to a varied environment. Rabbits will jump and therefore any furniture in the room will be used by them as an assault course – do not expect them to stay off the furniture. Most rabbits will happily play with their owners; however, owners need to be aware of the fear response and recognise whether the rabbit is happy or not. Provision of bolt-holes by way of cardboard boxes or tubes positioned around the house is one way of knowing whether the rabbit is happy or not. When the rabbit has had enough then they will take cover.

Most activity is seen in the early morning or late afternoon/early evening as with wild rabbits. During the middle of the day they are often resting.

### 5.1.5 Gnawing

Rabbits will gnaw their surroundings as part of their natural behaviour, and to wear down their teeth, and this needs to be taken into account for both outdoor and indoor rabbits. Outdoors the hutch and run needs to be made of a material that can be safely chewed. Wood should not be painted or varnished as these coatings can be ingested by the rabbit and may prove toxic or irritant. Structures also need to be sturdy enough to withstand chewing.

Indoor items that the owner does not wish to be chewed should be placed out of reach of the rabbit. Cables are one of the favourite things for rabbits to chew and obviously present a health risk to both the rabbits and the owners. Wherever possible, cables should be kept out of reach of rabbits. Where this is not possible, they should be covered with a casing that is difficult to chew or raised up out of reach of the rabbit. As chewing is a natural behaviour, the provision of things for the rabbit to chew will help. Hard food items such as carrots and wooden toys can be provided, although it is possible that the rabbit may prefer to chew more valuable objects.

### 5.1.6 Fear responses

If the rabbit is scared at any time then it will demonstrate a variety of responses. This may present as a rabbit which crouches low to the ground, ears flat to the head and not moving or a rabbit which demonstrates the fight or flight response. If the rabbit does not run away to hide in a bolt-hole, then it may thump with its hind feet to alert other rabbits of a problem, or may rarely vocalise, grunting or squeaking and bite or attack the problem with its front feet.

### 5.1.7 Interaction with others

Rabbits are social and will interact with other animals. In some cases it is possible for rabbits to happily get on with cats or even dogs. However, it is possible for rabbits to show aggression towards other animals, even dogs much bigger than themselves. Rabbits of the same sex may fight when kept together; however, if they are introduced to each other at a young age or allowed enough space to get away from each other, then it is possible for them to get along.

Rabbits are often kept with guinea pigs and whilst this is possible, it should be remembered that guinea pigs have different dietary requirements to rabbits and that rabbits can carry *Bordetella* sp. bacteria that can cause life-threatening disease in guinea pigs. For these reasons it is not always advisable to encourage the two species to be kept together.

### 5.1.8 Normal sexual activity

Sexually mature female rabbits show several normal patterns of sexual behaviour during the breeding season. Some of these behaviours are listed in Table 5.1. Sexually mature female rabbits may become aggressive towards their owners during periods of oestrus. Sexually mature male rabbits will often become aggressive towards other males, which they see as competitor, or may take out their frustration on other animals caged with them such as the unfortunate guinea pig. This is another reason for not housing guinea pigs with rabbits.

It is worth noting that even neutered female rabbits will mount each other from time to time. Neutered male rabbits will also mount each other but this occurs less often.

**Table 5.1** Normal sexual behaviour of the domestic rabbit

| Behaviour | Notes |
| --- | --- |
| Aggression | Mature males (this can be as early as 4 months of age) are territorial and will fight, often even if they have been kept together since kits. This will be exacerbated in the presence of a sexually active female rabbit |
| Circling | Does will often circle the male or their owner when in heat. Males may also circle the object of their affections and may make a low humming noise while they do so (Walshaw, 2006) |
| Lordosis | The doe will often adopt the lordotic posture, which is where she lies in sternal recumbency with the pelvis raised and the mid-lumbar region dipped ventrally, when in heat |
| Mounting behaviour | Sexually mature female rabbits will mount each other when in heat if kept in an all-female group – the dominant in-heat female does the mounting. The male rabbit will of course mount the female rabbit to allow mating to occur. He also bites the doe's neck during the short mating process and often emits a cry when he dismounts |
| Nest building | Female rabbits will nest build during pseudopregnancy by pulling fur out from her ventrum to make a nest and by chewing more items in her environment |
| Scent marking | Chin rubbing is often performed by sexually mature rabbits (especially males) as a means of territory marking as there are scent glands distributed along the line of the lower jaw |
| Urine spraying | Males and females will spray urine, often the male spraying onto the female in heat or onto a territory marker. However, males tend to do this more often and it is frequently associated with territory marking when they achieve sexual maturity |

If intending to breed domestic rabbits, it is advised to introduce the females to the males as females are surprisingly more territorial than the bucks. Alternatively, they may both be introduced into a neutral territory for mating. Females are generally bred from the age of 5–6 months.

## 5.2 Problems and possible solutions

### 5.2.1 Introducing a new rabbit

Introducing a new adult male rabbit to another adult male rabbit is very difficult as they are very likely to fight. If males (even castrated ones) are to be kept together successfully, they should be introduced before sexual maturity (i.e. before at least 5–6 months of age and preferably before 4 months). In addition, if a rabbit is debilitated or has been used to living on its own for some time, it is generally not advised to introduce a new rabbit to its environment.

If it is necessary to introduce two adult female rabbits for the first time or an adult male and adult female, then it is best to make sure they are both neutered if possible. They should be introduced together in a large open space with no hutches/hides but some favourite food items and rabbit suitable toys/obstacles. The two rabbits are introduced to this area and closely watched. They will be naturally suspicious of each other at first and may rush up to each other and then rush away again. Providing no serious biting or scratching occurs, leave the two together.

When it comes time to house them, they should then be housed separately for the night and reintroduced into the neutral territory again the following day. This may need to be repeated for 7–10 days before they are content enough and safe enough to be left together overnight. Whether this is possible is assessed by the observation of the two rabbits lying quietly side by side in the neutral territory. At this point the two may then be transferred to the hutch and locked in together for a few minutes again under close observation. If this results in no fighting they may be shut into the hutch for a few hours during the day while someone is around to watch over them. If all goes well, the rabbits may then be locked in overnight.

## 5.2.2 Chewing/gnawing

Preventing gnawing of household items is extremely difficult, and electric cables in particular, which may harm the rabbit, should be elevated out of the way or encased in a protective guard sheath to prevent potential electrocution incidents. Rabbits are designed to gnaw and so breaking this behaviour completely is not possible.

It may be possible to dissuade some rabbits from gnawing specific items such as carpets and skirting boards. As the rabbit starts to gnaw, a sharp 'No' followed either by walking towards the rabbit (which makes it think you are going to pick it up) or by squirting the rabbit with a small amount of tap water in a water pistol often stops the activity. When the rabbit stops gnawing, stop walking towards/squirting water at him/her and eventually the majority of rabbits associate the mildly aversive response with gnawing that part of the furniture/room and so cease this activity. In addition, the provision of material such as cardboard tubes, carrots or other safe, hard vegetables for the rabbit to gnaw and destroy may also deflect some of this natural activity away from the house.

### 5.2.3 Urine spraying and faecal marking

Both of these activities are commoner in all male sexually mature rabbits than neutered ones. To reduce the likelihood of these activities, neutering at 5–6 months of age is recommended. In addition, maintaining a stable pattern of feeding and husbandry can add to the avoidance of stress and so demonstration of such behaviour.

### 5.2.4 Aggression and fear

This is most commonly associated with all female sexually mature rabbits during the breeding season, although males will also be strongly territorial and is generally directed towards the owner. In these cases neutering can be beneficial.

However, aggression can have many causes including fear response, poor socialisation, disease processes and pain. A thorough veterinary examination may yield more information regarding disease and pain such as spinal arthritis, for example. If the aggression occurs during manipulation of an area of spondylosis, or if the rabbit is picked up roughly, then an aggressive response is understandable.

Some rabbits 'discover' that aggression towards their owner when he or she attempts to pick them up leads to the desired result – i.e. the owner does not try to pick them up again. In these cases persistence is the key and regular attempts to pick the rabbit up (if necessary with extra layers of clothing on to avoid bites or by first throwing a towel over the rabbit to aid handling) should be made until the rabbit realises that such behaviour does not allow it to get its own way.

It may be possible to win over a rabbit with repeated hand-feeding of favourite treats over a period of several weeks. This should be done without any other activity which may induce fear or aggression in the rabbit. Eventually, the majority of rabbits will associate the owner's hand with food and approach the owner when he or she enters the cage. It may be possible to slowly stroke the rabbit around the head and dorsum, either with the bare hand or if the rabbit has bitten the owner in the past, then using a plastic rod or wooden spoon.

Aggression between rabbits is often associated with hierarchical dominance. This sort of behaviour does not respond well to surgical neutering (unlike aggression towards owners), as a hierarchy must be formed irrespective of the reproductive status of the rabbits. If a stable hierarchy (i.e. one in which fighting is minimal/absent) is created within a few days to a week or so, then the owner need not intervene (except in severe attacks). However, if the group continues to fight (often there is one outcast rabbit) then sadly the removal of the most put-upon rabbit may be necessary for its own health and safety.

## 5.2.5 Demonstration of pain

Rabbits are very poor at demonstrating pain. Their natural response is to become quieter, less active and often to reduce or stop eating and performing caecotrophy. These are subtle signs often in the face of quite serious pain, but it is a survival tactic as rabbits are a prey species. A wild rabbit which was obviously injured or in pain would be easy prey for a predator and likely to be selected out of a group of others. Covering up pain makes this less likely but also makes it very difficult for the nurse and vet to spot when a rabbit is actually suffering. Only by monitoring carefully the features above such as food intake, activity levels and faecal pellet/caecotroph output is it often possible to detect the signs of discomfort and pain. Very occasionally some rabbits will vocalise when in pain. In the author's experience this is often associated with intense visceral pain such as pyelonephritis/renoliths or gastrointestinal tract bloat. Teeth grinding (bruxism) can also be another inconsistent clinical sign of discomfort.

## 5.2.6 Breakdown in toilet training

This most commonly occurs due to stress and fear in the pet rabbit, particularly if they feel their litter tray is in a location that is too busy (Magnus, 2005). In these instances, removing the source of the upheaval such as an additional pet cat or dog from the room where the rabbit's tray is kept may work. Alternatively, let the rabbit decide where it wishes to urinate/defaecate and then move the tray to that area. It is also advisable not to change the litter used in the tray. Expandable cat litter should not be used as rabbits may eat this and develop impactions, but substrates such as shavings/sawdust or hay/straw may be preferable.

## 5.2.7 Self-mutilation

This is uncommon in rabbits but has been reported (Rees-Davies, 2003). It is where a rabbit attacks itself, usually a distal limb, causing often severe self-trauma. It may be associated with stress and boredom, pain (whether direct or referred or neural pain) and a fungal contamination of food (ergot poisoning). In addition, there is some evidence that this behaviour may have a genetic component as certain family lines have shown a predisposition to the problem. It is necessary to rule out other possible causes such as an allergic skin problem, a subcutaneous foreign body such as a grass seed or neoplasia amongst others. However, once diagnosed it can be a challenge to treat. Non-steroidal anti-inflammatory drugs such as meloxicam have been used, along with behavioural modifiers. In addition, if it is thought to be associated with boredom, the introduction of new toys or hiding favourite food items around the house/cage for the rabbit to explore and find may help.

## Sources of further information

The Association of Pet Behaviour – http://www.apbc.org
Rabbit Behaviour Advisory Group – http://www.rabbitbehaviour.co.uk
Rabbit Welfare Association & Fund – http://www.rabbitwelfare.co.uk

## References

Jezierski, T., Mekking, P. and Wiepkema, P.R. (1993) Handling and diet-induced atherosclerosis in rabbits. *Laboratory Animals* 27:235–239.

Kersten, A.M.P., Meijsser, F.M. and Metx, J.H.M. (1989) Effects of early handling on later open field behaviour in rabbits. *Applied Animal Behaviour Science* 24: 157–167.

Magnus, E. (2005) Behaviour of the pet rabbits: what is normal and why do problems develop? *Journal of Veterinary Postgraduate Study in Practice* 27:531–535.

Rees-Davies, R. (2003) Self-mutilation in rabbits. *New Direction* January 2003, p. 13.

Walshaw, S.O. (2006) Behaviour problems. In: *BSAVA Manual of Rabbit Medicine and Surgery*, 2nd edn (eds, Meredith, A. and Flecknell, P.), BSAVA, Gloucestershire, pp. 137–143.

## Further reading

McBride, A., Magnus, E. and Hearne, G. (2004) Behaviour problems in the domestic rabbit. In: *The APBC Book of Companion Animal Behaviour* (ed., Appleby, D.), Souvenir Press, London.

# Restraint, Handling, Anaesthesia, Analgesia and Fluid Therapy

## 6.1 Restraint and handling

### 6.1.1 Do we need to restrain the rabbit patient?

There are some general guidelines to follow before restraint is attempted in order to safeguard the rabbit's welfare.

These points include the following:

1. Is the patient severely debilitated and in respiratory distress?
   Examples include the pneumonic rabbit, with obvious oculonasal discharge and dyspnoea. Excessive or rough handling of these patients is contraindicated.
2. Is the animal docile?
   Examples of aggressive animals could be poorly handled house rabbits, some male rabbits during the breeding season and female rabbits with young.
3. Is the rabbit suffering from metabolic bone disease?
   This is often seen in young rabbits. The diet may have been inadequate with regard to calcium and vitamin D3 and exposure to natural sunlight may be absent particularly in house rabbits, hence long bone mineralisation during growth will be poor leading to spontaneous/ easily fractured bones.
4. Does the rabbit patient require medication/physical examination?
   If so restraint may be essential but the above points should still be considered and appropriate medical precautions taken as well as minimising the stress involved.

## 6.1.2 Handling techniques

The majority of domestic rabbits are docile, but the odd aggressive doe or buck, usually those not used to being handled, does exist. In rabbits the main dangers to the handler are from the claws, which can inflict deep scratches, and the incisors, which can produce deep bites. Aggression is frequently worst at the start of the breeding season in March/April or when the rabbit is frightened. In addition to the damage they may cause the handler, a struggling rabbit may lash out with its powerful hindlimbs and fracture or dislocate its spine. Severe stress can also be associated with cardiac failure in some individuals. Rapid and safe restraint is therefore essential.

If aggressive, the rabbit may be grasped by the scruff with one hand whilst the other supports underneath the rear legs. If the rabbit is not aggressive then one hand may be placed under the thorax, with the thumb and first two fingers encircling the front limbs, whilst the other is placed under the rear legs to support the back, the dorsum of the rabbit being held against the handler's stomach/chest (see Fig. 6.5).

When transferred from one room to another, the rabbit must be held close to the handler's body. Non-fractious individuals may also be supported with their heads pushed into the crook of one arm, with that forearm supporting the length of the rabbit's ventral body and the other hand then used to place pressure/grasp the scruff region (see Figs 6.1–6.4).

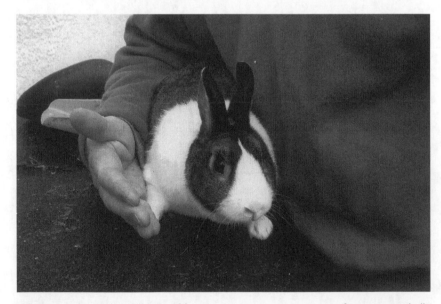

**Figure 6.1** Steady rabbit on table prior to restraining. Courtesy of Fiona Campbell.

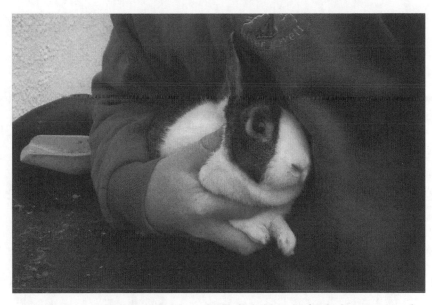

**Figure 6.2** Hold the rabbit close to the body, holding the forelimbs. Courtesy of Fiona Campbell.

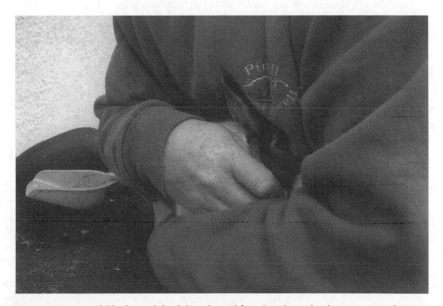

**Figure 6.3** Hold limbs with both hands and face head into body. Courtesy of Fiona Campbell.

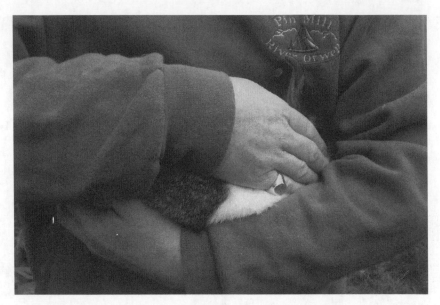

**Figure 6.4** Lift rabbit supporting ventrum and hindlimbs. Courtesy of Fiona Campbell.

Once caught, the rabbit may be calmed further by wrapping him or her in a towel, similar to the method used for cats, so that just the head/ears protrude. There are also specific rabbit papooses encircling the rabbit, but leaving the head and ears free. This allows ear blood sampling and oral examinations, but controls their hindlimbs in particular, preventing lashing out and possible injury to handler and rabbit alike. It is important not to allow them to overheat in this position, as rabbits do not have significant sweat glands and do not actively pant. They can therefore quickly overheat if their environmental temperature exceeds 23–25°C with potentially fatal results.

*Trancing*

This is a technique for inducing tonic immobility or a 'trance-like' state in rabbits by placing them on their backs. The rabbit is tilted slightly head downwards and held in this position for 2–3 minutes gently stroking the pectoral area. In some cases it may allow positioning for ventrodorsal X-rays, for nail clipping and examination of the incisor teeth (Malley, 2007). However, it may be a very stressful procedure in some individual rabbits and so should be used with care and obviously not used for any potentially painful procedure. The rabbit should also not be left

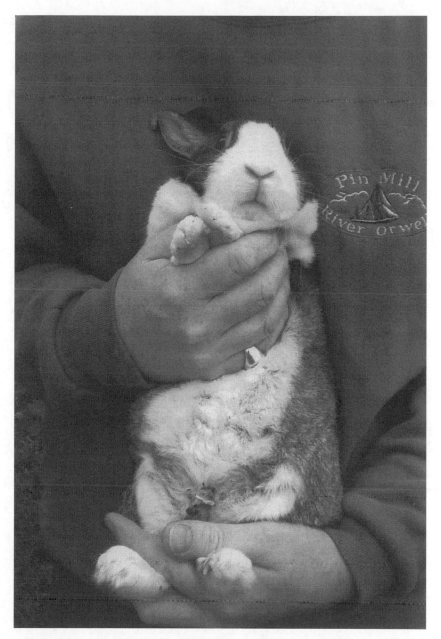

**Figure 6.5**   Restraint of the rabbit to allow examination of ventrum, supporting weight. Courtesy of Fiona Campbell.

unattended whilst in the trance. Recovery is made by simply returning the rabbit to ventral recumbency.

## 6.2 Anaesthesia

### 6.2.1 Introduction

Anaesthesia may be necessary for a number of reasons in rabbits:

- For sample collection, such as blood testing or urine collection, particularly in fractious animals
- For procedures such as radiography
- For oral examinations
- For surgical procedures

Anaesthetic procedures are now becoming routine for rabbits. The improved levels of success in this area have been mainly due to our awareness of certain problems which frequently beset these patients such as a high prevalence of low-grade respiratory infections. It is therefore vitally important to make an assessment as to whether or not the patient is fit to allow chemical restraint to occur.

Factors which have to be considered prior to the anaesthesia of rabbits are the following:

### *Low-grade respiratory infections*

Many rabbits suffer from low-grade levels of respiratory infection all of their lives. Some will cope with this on a day-to-day basis, but when anaesthetised, the respiratory rate slows, and respiratory secretions, already thickened/increased due to the chronic infections, become more tenacious and physical blockage of the airways can occur with resulting hypoxaemia.

### *Respiratory system anatomy*

Rabbits are obligate nose breathers, with their soft palates permanently locked around the epiglottis. Hence, if the patient has a blocked nose, whether that be due to pus, blood, tumours or abscesses, then respiratory arrest is made much more likely under anaesthetic induction or where no intubation is performed.

*Hypothermia*

Due to their relatively small size and large body surface areas to volume ratios, particularly in the dwarf breeds, rabbits are prone to hypothermia during anaesthesia. This is due to the cooling effect of the inhaled gases and reduced muscular activity. It is dangerous to place a patient already hypothermic through an anaesthetic without reversing this change.

*Dehydration*

Respiratory fluid loses during the drying gaseous anaesthetic procedures are much greater than in cats, dogs or larger species. Hence, placing a dehydrated rabbit patient through an anaesthetic without prior fluid therapy is also dangerous.

## 6.2.2 Preoperative checks

*Weight measurement*

This is vitally important to be accurate. A mistake of just 50–100 g in a dwarf Netherland say will lead to an under-/overdosage of 10%. The use of scales which will read accurately down to at least 10 g in weight is therefore essential.

*Blood biochemistry and haematology testing*

This is starting to become much more common in rabbits, and should be considered in every clinically unwell or senior patient (rabbits over 4 years of age) where a large enough sample may be obtained.

The lateral ear vein may be used with a 25- to 27-gauge needle (Fig. 6.6). The prior application of a local anaesthetic cream (e.g. EMLA®) to the site and the warming of the ear under a heat lamp/hot water bottle are advised to allow dilation of the vessel. Alternatively, the cephalic vein, saphenous vein (Fig. 6.7) or the jugular vein may be used. The latter should be used with caution as it is the only source of blood drainage from the eyes, and so if a thrombus forms in this vessel, ocular oedema and permanent damage or even loss of the eye may occur.

*Fasting*

Rabbits do not need to be fasted prior to being anaesthetised, as they have a very tight cardiac sphincter at the top of the stomach, preventing

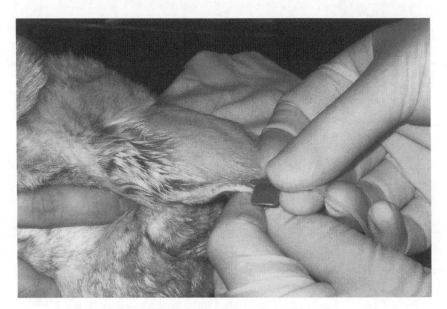

**Figure 6.6** Placement of butterfly catheter in lateral ear vein.

vomiting. Indeed, starving may actually be deleterious to the patient's health as it causes a cessation in gut contractility and subsequent ileus. It is important, however, to ensure that no food is present in the mouth at the time of induction, which may impede intubation or become inhaled, hence a period of 30–60 minutes starvation is used.

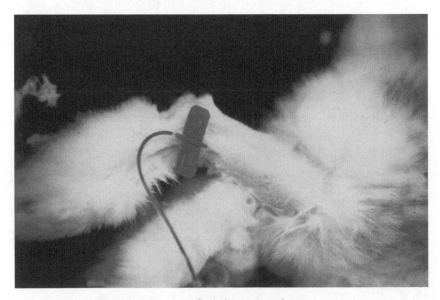

**Figure 6.7** Butterfly catheter in saphenous vein.

## 6.2.3 Preoperative medication ('pre-meds')

So-called 'pre-meds' are used because they either provide a smooth induction/recovery to anaesthesia or because they ensure a reduction of airway secretions, act as a respiratory stimulant, or prevent serious bradycardia.

### Anti-muscarinics

Doses of 0.05 mg/kg atropine sulphate have been used subcutaneously 30 minutes before induction to help prevent excessive bradycardia which often occurs during the induction phase. However, it is not so useful in rabbits as in other mammals as around 60% of rabbits have a serum atropinesterase which breaks down atropine before it has a chance to work.

Therefore, glycopyrrolate, which functions in a similar manner to atropine, may also be used at doses of 0.01 mg/kg subcutaneously and this is not affected by the serum atropinesterases.

In both cases there is concern that anti-muscarinics increase the viscosity of respiratory tract secretions, and this may lead to blockage of smaller airways or endotracheal tubes. This author routinely does not use anti-muscarinics for this reason, although glycopyrrolate is an essential component of any emergency/crash kit for rabbits (see Chapter 10).

### Tranquillisers

Tranquillisers are frequently used to reduce the stress of induction in mammals. Rabbits will breath-hold during gaseous induction to the point where they become cyanotic. In rabbits, the 'shock' organ is the lungs, and during intense stress the pulmonary circulation can go into spasm, making the hypoxia due to breath-holding even worse, even to the point of collapse and cardiac arrest.

Acepromazine can be used at doses of 0.1–0.5 mg/kg in rabbits. In general, it is a very safe premedicant even in debilitated animals. It can, however, prolong the recovery time as there is no reversal agent. This may cause problems with gut stasis in some individuals as they do not eat rapidly postoperatively. In addition, it should not be used in dehydrated individuals or those with cardiac disturbances.

### Neuroleptanalgesics

Fentanyl/fluanisone combination (Hypnorm®) may be used at varying doses as either a premedicant, a sedative, or as part of an injectable full anaesthesia. As a premedicant, doses of 0.1 mL/kg for rabbits can produce sufficient sedation to prevent breath-holding and allow gaseous induction. The dose is given intramuscularly 15–20 minutes before induction. Hypnorm® is an irritant and large doses in one spot may cause postoperative lameness. It can be partially reversed with butorphanol at 0.2 mg/kg intravenously, or buprenorphine at 0.05 mg/kg, both of which are partial opioid agonists and so will reverse the full opioid agonist fentanyl.

Fluid therapy is also a vitally important pre-anaesthetic consideration and is mentioned later in this chapter.

## 6.2.4 Induction of anaesthesia

*Injectable agents*

Table 6.1 outlines some of the advantages and disadvantages of injectable anaesthetics in rabbits. It should be noted that there is increasing evidence that different strains/breeds of rabbits respond differently to anaesthetics. In particular, one study has shown how two different strains of domestic rabbit responded differently to the same injectable anaesthetics – notably propofol, medetomidine and ketamine (Avsaroglu *et al.*, 2003).

**Propofol**

In rabbits apnoea can be a problem. If given slowly intravenously at 3–10 mg/kg, propofol can be used as an induction agent, but intubation should be performed as intermittent positive pressure ventilation may need to be instituted should apnoea occur.

**Dissociative anaesthetics (ketamine) and alpha-2 agonist combinations**

Ketamine can be used at a dose of 15 mg/kg in conjunction with medetomidine at 0.25 mg/kg or with xylazine at 5 mg/kg (Flecknall, 2000). The

**Table 6.1** Advantages and disadvantages of injectable anaesthetics

| Advantages | Disadvantages |
|---|---|
| Easily administered | Delay in reversal |
| Minimal stress | Hypoxia and hypotension common |
| Prevent breath-holding | Tissue necrosis |
| Inexpensive | Organ metabolism required in many cases |

advantage is a quick and stress-free anaesthetic, but the combination will cause blueing of the membranes and make detection of hypoxia difficult. Respiratory depression during longer procedures may become a problem and intubation is often advised.

A so-called triple combination of 5 mg/kg ketamine with 0.05 mg/kg medetomidine and 0.5 mg/kg butorphanol can also be used intravenously to induce and provide a short-duration general anaesthetic. This minimises the individual doses of the drugs and yet provides sufficient depth of anaesthesia for minor dental work, radiography, etc. The addition of butorphanol to ketamine and medetomidine combinations increases the duration of anaesthesia but also can slightly increase the degree of respiratory depression (Hedenqvist *et al.*, 2002). For more advanced surgical procedures it is advisable to intubate the rabbit and maintain on oxygen and isoflurane or oxygen and sevoflurane.

Alternatively, the 'triple' combination may be given subcutaneously at 10 mg/kg ketamine plus 0.2 mg/kg medetomidine and 0.5 mg/kg butorphanol. This method takes 10–15 minutes to take effect and again requires intubation and oxygen plus isoflurane or oxygen plus sevoflurane for the majority of surgical procedures.

Studies in the rabbit have shown that administration of medetomidine/ketamine combinations via the subcutaneous route produced equivalent effects to those induced by administering it via the intramuscular route (Hedenqvist *et al.*, 2002).

In all cases when using injectable anaesthetics it is advisable to provide 100% oxygen either via intubation or a face mask to minimise the hypoxia which can result, particularly when using triple combinations, in increased levels of respiratory depression.

The medetomidine in any case may be reversed using atipamazole at 1 mg/kg to speed up postoperative recovery.

### Fentanyl/fluanisone (Hypnorm®)

This drug combination is a neuroleptanalgesic licensed for use in rabbits in the UK. Fentanyl is a morphine/opioid derivative, and fluanisone is the neuroleptic.

Sedation is produced at doses of 0.5 mL/kg intramuscularly. This produces sedation and immobilisation for 30–60 minutes, but its analgesic effect due to the opioid derivative fentanyl will persist for some time after. It may, however, be reversed with 0.5 mg/kg butorphanol intravenously or 0.05 mg/kg buprenorphine, both of which will counteract the fentanyl and its analgesia and substitute their own pain relief.

Alternatively to provide anaesthetic depth, fentanyl/fluanisone may be combined with diazepam (0.3 mL Hypnorm® to 2 mg/kg diazepam) intraperitoneally, or intravenously (but in separate syringes as they do not mix), or with midazolam (0.3 mL Hypnorm® to 2 mg/kg midazolam) intramuscularly or intraperitoneally in the same syringe. Alternatively, Hypnorm® may be given intramuscularly first and then 15 minutes later the midazolam may be given intravenously into the lateral ear vein. These two combinations provide good analgesia and muscle relaxation with induction and duration of anaesthesia of 20–40 minutes.

The fentanyl portion may be reversed again with buprenorphine or butorphanol given intravenously, or in emergencies the drug naloxone at 0.1 mg/kg intramuscularly or intravenously may be given, but this provides no substitute analgesia.

Fentanyl/fluanisone combinations are generally well tolerated in most rabbits, but they can produce respiratory depression and hypoxia.

### Gaseous agents

Table 6.2 gives some advantage and disadvantages of gaseous anaesthetics in rabbits.

### Halothane

In general, induction concentrations should not exceed 3%, and anaesthesia can usually be maintained with 1.5% halothane in 100% oxygen.

Halothane has disadvantages in that it can induce cardiac arrhythmias, particularly in rabbits, and induce profound breath-holding. It is more likely to induce an adrenaline surge during induction in rabbits than isoflurane and so more likely to exacerbate any cardiovascular problems (Gonzalez *et al.*, 2005). Its use in small mammals with hepatic disease should be avoided due to its metabolism by the liver. For

**Table 6.2**  Advantages and disadvantages of gaseous anaesthetics

| Advantages | Disadvantages |
| --- | --- |
| Faster alteration of depth of anaesthesia possible | Increased drying effect on respiratory membranes |
| Recovery times shorter | Hypothermic effect from above |
| Less organ metabolism (for some, e.g. isoflurane and sevoflurane) | Difficulty in induction as rabbits can breath-hold |

these reasons it is generally not advised to use halothane to anaesthetise rabbits.

### Isoflurane

This is now becoming the most widespread used gas for maintenance and indeed induction and is licensed for use in rabbits in the UK. Usually, premedication is used to prevent breath-holding and to provide analgesia as once recovered from the anaesthetic, isoflurane does not provide any residual analgesia. Its outweighing advantages though are in its safety for the debilitated patient as <0.3% of the gas is metabolised hepatically, the rest merely being exhaled for recovery to occur. Recovery is therefore rapid and its minimum alveolar concentration (MAC) is 2.05%. However, during the recovery phase there is a greater increase in adrenaline with isoflurane than with halothane, and so care should be taken to look out in the immediate post-anaesthetic phase for cardiac disturbances (Adams *et al.*, 1991).

Induction levels vary at 2.5–4% and maintenance usually is 1.5–2.5% in 100% oxygen, assuming adequate analgesia. Breath-holding can still occur even with premedication, but the practice of supplying 100% oxygen to the patient for 2 minutes prior to anaesthetic administration helps minimise hypoxia. Isoflurane is then gradually introduced, first 0.5% for 2 minutes, then on assuming regular breathing, increase to 1% for 2 minutes, and so on, until anaesthetic levels are reached – allowing a smooth induction.

### Sevoflurane

Sevoflurane is generally better tolerated than isoflurane in rabbits. There is less breath-holding as it is less irritant on the mucous membranes and therefore induction is smoother and quicker than isoflurane. It has a minimum alveolar concentration of 3.7% (Scheller *et al.*, 1988). At high induction concentrations, as have been advocated in some instances for cats and dogs (i.e. 7–8% sevoflurane), rabbits will still breath-hold. Therefore, this author finds that induction levels of 3–4% sevoflurane in 100% oxygen are sufficient to provide a relatively quick induction with minimal breath-holding. As with isoflurane there is no residual analgesia after recovery; therefore, pre-anaesthetic and post-anaesthetic analgesia is required where noxious procedures are performed.

Recovery from anaesthesia is quicker than isoflurane and it is minimally metabolised by the liver.

## 6.2.5 Maintenance of anaesthesia

*Intubation*

As with all gaseous anaesthetics the placement of an endotracheal tube after induction for maintenance is to be recommended whenever possible.

In rabbits the use of a number 1 Wisconsin flat bladed paediatric laryngoscope and a 2- to 3-mm tube is advised (Flecknell, 1991). The rabbit is first induced with either an injectable anaesthetic or face masked with an inhalational one. It is then placed in dorsal recumbency, allowing the larynx to fall dorsally and into view. A rabbit mouth gag aids visibility at this stage, and the laryngoscope and endotracheal tube are inserted pulling the tongue out and to one side of the mouth. A guide wire may first be used to pass through the laryngeal opening, and once in, the endotracheal tube is threaded over the top, and the wire withdrawn.

Alternatively the rabbit may be intubated blindly. This is performed in sternal recumbency after initial induction. The head is lifted vertically off the table with one hand and the ET tube inserted with the other, midline orally until slight resistance and a cough is elicited. It is then advanced slowly, and air passage checked through the tube to ensure correct placement.

In rabbits the use of a local anaesthetic (e.g. xylocaine) spray on the larynx or the end of the ET tube is useful to reduce laryngospasm and aid intubation.

*Intermittent positive pressure ventilation*

This may be necessary in some individuals who proceed to breath-hold during induction. Intubation is preferred as complete control over flow rates and frequency are possible. The anaesthetist should aim to produce a cycle of 6–12 breaths before pausing to check respiration and if required to perform cardiac massage.

If intubation is not possible then four options are available:

1. To ensure a tight-fitting face mask and have an Ayres T-piece/ Mapleson C (Fig. 6.8)/modified Bain circuit with half litre bag attached, which can be used to attempt ventilation.
2. To place a nasopharyngeal tube via the medial meatus of the nose into the pharyngeal area. Then to supply 4 L or so of oxygen (to combat the resistance of the small diameter tubing of 1–2 mm) via this route.

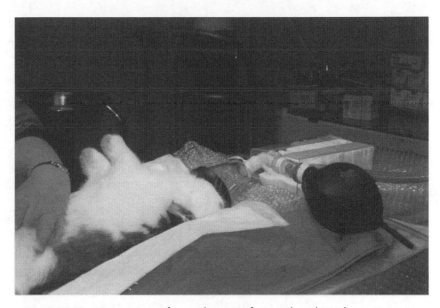

**Figure 6.8** Maintenance of anaesthesia via face mask and Mapleson C circuit.

3. Perform an emergency tracheostomy with a 25-/27-gauge needle attached to the oxygen outlet, placing the needle in between the laryngeal C-shaped supporting cartilages ventrally. Alternatively, a specifically designed or adapted Teflon® catheter with a Luer adaptor may be inserted in a similar manner (see Chapter 10).
4. In addition, there is another option if direct intubation is not possible – that of the 'laryngeal mask'. This is the use of a human paediatric laryngeal mask, which is basically an endotracheal tube, with an inflatable cuff at its tip that acts like a small mask to sit over the laryngeal inlet. The tube is inserted through the mouth so the tip sits in the caudal pharyngeal area and the cuff is then inflated to block off the oral and nasal cavity communication with the larynx. A study has shown that this technique is preferable to face mask inhalation, but that if intermittent positive pressure ventilation is used then gastric tympany is a possibility (Bateman *et al.*, 2003). However, if voluntary respiration occurs, then gas exchange has been shown to be comparable to endotracheal intubation (Cruz *et al.*, 2000).

*Anaesthetic circuits used*

For rabbits less than 2 kg in weight, a modified Bain or Mapleson C circuit is the best one to use for removing as much of the dead space as is possible (Girling, 2003). For larger rabbits in the 2–10 kg range, an Ayres T-piece is usually sufficient.

## 6.2.6 Supportive therapy during and after anaesthesia

*Recumbency*

During most surgical procedures the method of restraint/recumbency will be dependent on the area being operated on. A lot of routine procedures such as castration and spaying operations require the patient to be placed in dorsal recumbency. This creates some problems for rabbits as they have developed an enlarged hindgut, which can place more weight on the diaphragm, and so more resistance to inspiration. During lengthy surgical procedures this may lead to apnoea and hypoxia. Placement therefore with the cranial end of the patient elevated above the caudal when in dorsal recumbency can improve this situation by allowing the gut to fall away from the diaphragm.

*Maintenance of body temperature*

Maintenance of core body temperature is vitally important in all patients to ensure successful recovery from anaesthesia, but is particularly important in small mammals such as rabbits. This is primarily due to their increased surface area in relation to their volume, so allowing more heat to escape per gram of animal. To help minimise this the following actions may be taken:

1. Perform minimal surgical scrubbing of the site and minimal clipping of fur from the area. Do not use surgical spirit as this rapidly cools the skin.
2. Ensure the room temperature is at the warm end of comfortable.
3. Place the patient onto either a water circulating heat pad, a hot air circulating blanket, or use latex gloves/hot water bottles filled with warm water around the patient (making sure that the patient does not directly contact with the containers as skin burns may ensue).
4. Administer warmed isotonic fluids subcutaneously/intravenously/intraperitoneally during and prior to surgery.

It is also worth noting that anaesthetic gases have a rapidly cooling effect on the oral and respiratory membranes, and so patients maintained on gaseous anaesthetics will cool down quicker than those on injectable ones, and this will worsen as the length of the anaesthesia increases.

These actions will prevent hypothermia setting in and so improve anaesthesia success rates. It is worth noting, however, that hyperthermia may be as bad as hypothermia. Rabbits generally have few or no sweat glands, and so heat cannot be lost via this route. A rectal thermometer is useful to monitor body temperature, which should be between 37°C and 39.4°C in the domestic rabbit.

### 6.2.7 Fluid therapy

*Assessment of dehydration and calculation of fluid volumes*

Intra-, pre- and postoperative fluid therapy is very important in rabbits, even for routine surgery. The small size and relatively large body surface area in relation to volume of these patients means that they will also dehydrate much faster, gram for gram, than a larger cat or dog. Studies have shown that the provision of maintenance levels of fluids to rabbits during and immediately after routine surgery improved anaesthetic safety levels by as much as 15% in some cases, with higher levels if the surgery was being performed on severely debilitated animals.

It is therefore to be strongly recommended that all small mammal patients receive fluids during and after an anaesthetic whether it be routine or not.

A lot of fluid intake is normally consumed as 'food', i.e. in the form of fresh vegetation. This is difficult to take into consideration, and therefore it is safer to assume that the debilitated rabbit will not be eating enough for this to matter in the calculation. Once it is appreciated that maintenance for rabbits is double that required for the average cat or dog (i.e. 80–100 mL/kg/day), then deficits may be calculated in the same manner as follows.

As with cats and dogs, assume that 1% dehydration equates with need to supply 10 mL/kg body weight fluid replacement in addition to the maintenance requirements.

Assumptions then have to be made on the degree of dehydration of the rabbit concerned (see Table 6.3).

Alternatively, if a blood sample may be obtained, a 1% increase in packed cell volume, associated with an increase in total proteins, may be assumed to equate to 10 mL/kg fluid deficit.

**Table 6.3** Degrees of dehydration assessment in the rabbit

| Level of dehydration | Clinical signs |
| --- | --- |
| 3–5% dehydrated | Increased thirst, slight lethargy, tacky mucous membranes |
| 7–10% dehydrated | Increased thirst leading to anorexia, dullness, tenting of the skin and slow return to normal, dry mucous membranes, 'dull corneas' |
| 10–15% dehydrated | Dull comatose, skin remains tented after pinching, desiccating mucous membranes |

If severe dehydration is present, postponement of anaesthesia and correction of the fluid deficit over 2–3 days should be considered, for example:

*Day 1:* Maintenance fluid levels + 50% of calculated dehydration factor.
*Day 2:* Maintenance fluid levels + 50% of calculated dehydration factor.
*Day 3:* Maintenance fluid levels.

### Routes of administration of fluids

This will depend to a certain extent on the severity of the dehydration.

### Subcutaneous

Routine short-duration anaesthetic procedures with little previous dehydration and no blood loss may simply need warmed isotonic subcutaneous fluids given over the lateral thorax and scruff region. The total volume should be divided up over multiple sites with a maximum volume of 2–3 mL in small rabbits and up to 10 mL in giant breeds at any one site.

### Intraperitoneal

For dehydration levels of 3% or thereabouts it may be sufficient to give hypotonic or isotonic fluids intraperitoneally. Care needs to be taken to avoid puncturing the capacious gut, and for this reason it is often recommended that the rabbit is placed in dorsal recumbency with the caudal body raised to allow the gut to fall away from the injection site, which is the lower right quadrant of the ventral abdomen, to one side of midline (Fig. 6.9). This method is therefore only regularly used immediately postoperatively when the rabbit is still partially/fully anaesthetised to minimise stress.

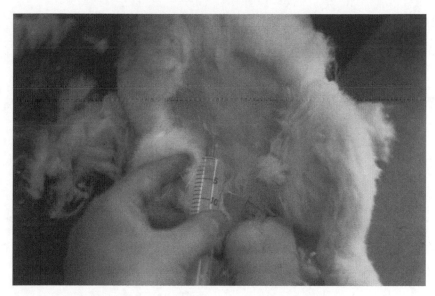

**Figure 6.9**   Intraperitoneal fluid administration. Reproduced with permission from the BSAVA *Textbook of Veterinary Nursing* (Lane, Cooper and Turner).

### Intravenous and intra-osseous

If dehydration levels exceed 3% then consideration should be given to intravenous or intra-osseous fluids.

The lateral ear vein is probably the easiest to use as an intravenous route. It can be catheterised as follows:

1. The area should be shaved and surgically prepared. Warm the ear under a lamp/hot water bottle or apply local anaesthetic cream to dilate vessel (NB: if the rabbit is sedated with Hypnorm, the ear veins will dilate anyway).
2. Use the lateral ear vein which runs along the most caudal/lateral margin of the pinna. Do not be tempted to use the apparently larger vessel that runs in the midline of the pinna as this is the central ear artery. Catheterisation of this vessel may lead to thrombosis followed by ear tip necrosis.
3. Use a 25- to 27-gauge butterfly catheter or latex over the needle catheter, preflushed with heparinised saline. Once in place, tape this in securely and reflush. Attach the intravenous drip tubing or catheter bung to the end of the butterfly catheter/latex catheter.
4. Apply an Elizabethan collar to the rabbit or intravenous drip guard to the intravenous tubing to prevent chewing and attach the

intravenous tubing to the syringe driver. It is possible to tape the butterfly catheter tubing to the back of the rabbit's head if using intermittent intravenous boluses, but it is important to ensure the catheter is regularly flushed with heparin/saline.

The cephalic vein may also be used as for the cat and dog, although this vein may be paired. A 25- to 27-gauge over the needle or butterfly catheter may be used for access and taped in as for cats and dogs.

For the saphenous vein it is best to use a 25- to 27-gauge butterfly catheter as it is relatively fragile. It runs over the lateral aspect of the hock.

All of these routes can be used for intravenous boluses of up to 10 mL for larger rabbits and 5 mL for smaller dwarf breeds, but for continuous therapy a syringe driver is required (Fig. 6.10).

For intra-osseous fluid administration the proximal femur is the easiest bone to use. Landmarks to aim for are the fossa between the hip joint and the greater trochanter. A 20- to 23-gauge hypodermic needle or spinal needle is used. Generally the procedure requires sedation, although deep infiltration of the subcutaneous tissues and muscles may be performed with lignocaine in debilitated rabbits where sedation may be dangerous.

The fur is clipped and the area is surgically prepared. The needle is screwed into position in the same direction as the long axis of the femur,

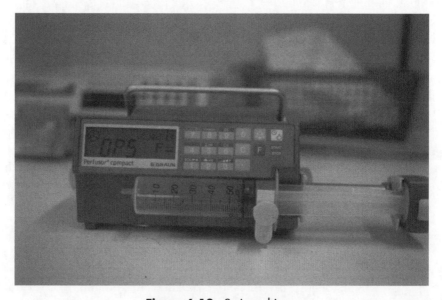

**Figure 6.10** Syringe driver.

a sudden pop being felt as the needle penetrates the marrow of the femur. It may be necessary to cut down through the skin with a sterile scalpel blade in some rabbits. This method will require a syringe driver perfusion device.

It is possible to use the proximal tibia but this is less well tolerated due to interference with the stifle joint. There is frequently a need for tubing guards or Elizabethan collars for all intravenous/intra-osseous techniques.

### Infusion devices

Due to their smaller size it is advisable when considering continuous infusion to use syringe drivers or infusion pumps capable of administering fluid rates down to 1 mL/hour. This is to avoid the inaccuracies inherent in drip sets which are magnified in smaller animals – either the rate is too fast and overperfusion occurs, or so slow that the catheter blocks.

## 6.2.8 Monitoring anaesthesia

### Reflexes

No one factor will allow you to assess anaesthetic depth. Indeed, in rabbits many of the useful techniques utilised in cats and dogs are not relevant. Eye position, for example, should not be used to assess depth of anaesthesia in rabbits. Instead, a useful method is to assess depth by the response to noxious stimuli such as limb pinch techniques.

Initially, though the first reflex lost is usually the righting reflex, the rabbit is unable to return to ventral recumbency.

The next reflex to be lost is the swallow reflex; however, this may be difficult to assess. Palpebral reflexes in dogs and cats (the response of blinking when the eye surface/cornea is lightly touched) are generally lost early on in the course of anaesthetic, but rabbits may retain this reflex until well into the deeper planes of surgical anaesthesia. The palpebral reflex is also altered by the anaesthetic agent chosen, with most inhalant gaseous anaesthetics causing loss of the reflex early on, but it is maintained with ketamine.

The pedal withdrawal reflex is useful in rabbits, being performed by extending the leg firmly pinching the toes. Loss of this reflex suggests surgical planes of anaesthesia, but rabbits again will retain the pedal reflex in the forelimbs until much deeper (and often dangerously deep) planes of anaesthesia are reached. Other pain stimuli such as the ear pinch are useful. Loss of this indicates a surgical plane of anaesthesia has been achieved.

### Cardiovascular monitoring

Monitoring of the heart and circulation may be performed in a conventional manner with stethoscope and femoral pulse evaluation or by oesophageal stethoscope. As with cats and dogs, increase in the respiratory and heart rates can be used to indicate lightening of the plane of anaesthesia. More sophisticated techniques may also be used with pulse oximetry to monitor heart rate and haemoglobin saturation. As with cats and dogs, the aim is to achieve 100% saturation and levels below 96% would indicate moderate-to-severe hypoxaemia, and the initiation of assisted ventilation below 92% would be potentially critical. The ear artery is useful for this in rabbits using a clip-on probe, conversely the linear probes may be used successfully on the ventral aspect of the tail against the coccygeal artery or again taped to the ear artery.

Electrocardiogram analysis may be performed using standard equipment. Changes in the polarity of the T-wave (either from negative to positive or vice versa) indicate hypoxia during anaesthesia. Profound bradycardia due to heart block is the commonest electrocardiogram abnormality, and if seen requires prompt treatment with anti-muscarinics such as glycopyrrolate and lightening or reversal of the anaesthesia.

Another extremely useful monitoring device is the Doppler probe which can detect blood flow in the smallest of vessels up to the heart itself. The Doppler probe converts blood flow into an audible sound through a speaker device, which can then be assessed by the anaesthetist during the surgery for changes in strength of the output and heart rates.

### Respiratory system monitoring

Respiratory monitors may also be used if the patient is intubated and many pulse oximeters have outlets for these, allowing assessment of respiratory rates. In addition, capnographs may be used in intubated rabbits to watch for hypoventilation and rebreathing. Obviously, these are not useful for patients which are being maintained on face masks or on injectable anaesthetics unless intubated.

## 6.3 Recovery and analgesia

### 6.3.1 Reversal of anaesthesia

Recovery from anaesthesia is improved with the use of suitable reversal agents if available. Examples include the use of atipamazole after medetomidine anaesthesia/sedation, and the use of naloxone, butorphanol or buprenorphine after opioid /Hypnorm® anaesthesia/sedation. Gaseous anaesthesia, particularly with isoflurane and sevoflurane, tends to result in more rapid recovery than the injectable anaesthetics, but all forms of anaesthesia recovery are improved by ensuring adequate maintenance of body temperature and hydration status during and after anaesthesia.

Most rabbits will benefit from a quiet darkened and warm room, allowing a controlled recovery. Subsequent fluid administration the same day is advisable as many of these patients will not be eating normally for the first 12–24 hours.

### 6.3.2 Analgesia

Analgesia is vitally important in the quick and smooth recovery process. Return to normal activity such as grooming, eating and drinking has been shown to be considerably shortened following adequate analgesia.

Analgesics frequently used in rabbits can be found in Table 6.4.

As with other mammals, the administration of analgesia prior to the onset of pain makes for the most effective control of pain. Analgesics are therefore frequently being used as part of premedication injections.

Choice of analgesic depends on the level of pain and other factors such as concurrent disease processes. Older non-steroidal anti-inflammatory

**Table 6.4** Analgesics used in small mammals

| Drug | Dosage | Frequency | Route |
|------|--------|-----------|-------|
| Butorphanol | 0.3 mg/kg | q4 hours | SC, IM, IV |
| Buprenorphine | 0.01–0.05 mg/kg | q8–12 hours | SC, IM, IV |
| Pethidine | 10 mg/kg | q2–3 hours | SC, IM |
| Carprofen | 1–4 mg/kg | q24 hours | PO, SC |
| Meloxicam | 0.3–0.6 mg/kg | q24 hours | PO, SC |

Information adapted from Flecknall (2006), Flecknall (1998) and Mason (1997).
q4 hours stands for 'every 4 hours', q8 hours for 'every 8 hours', and so on. PO, per os; IM, intramuscularly; SC, subcutaneously; IV, intravenously.
NB: None are licensed for use in rabbits in the UK.

**Table 6.5** Gut motility enhancing drugs for rabbits

| Drug | Dose rate | Frequency of dosing and notes |
| --- | --- | --- |
| Cisapride | 0.5 mg/kg PO | 12 hourly (now difficult to obtain) |
| Metoclopramide | 0.5 mg/kg SC | 8–12 hourly |
| Ranitidine | 2–5 mg/kg PO | 12 hourly (in combination with metoclopramide acts to promote motility as well as reducing acidity) |

NB: None are licensed for use in rabbits in the UK.

drugs such as flunixin, for example, are not good analgesics to use in dehydrated animals or those with renal disease; full-agonist opioids (e.g. morphine and pethidine) act to depress respiration and so may be contraindicated in severe respiratory disease cases.

### 6.3.3 Other postoperative supportive therapies

A rapid return to normal appetite is essential in rabbits to prevent postoperative complications such as intestinal ileus. This can be facilitated by ensuring good analgesia, adequate hydration and the use of reversible/quick recovery anaesthetics. In addition, providing the rabbit with a familiar foodstuff in its own bowl(s) is essential in many cases to reduce anxiety and rejection of food altogether. The patient may not be on the best diet for a rabbit when he or she comes into the surgery, but immediately after a surgical procedure and anaesthetic is not the time to start drastically altering it.

If dental surgery has been performed it may be necessary to hand-feed or syringe feed the rabbit with appropriate critical care and support formula diets (see Chapter 4). In addition, prokinetic drugs that stimulate gut motility and so help prevent ileus and encourage appetite can be used (see Table 6.5).

## References

Adams, H.A., Tengler, R. and Hempelmann, G. (1991) The stress reaction in the recovery phase from halothane and isoflurane anaesthesia. *Anaesthesist* 40:446–451.

Avsaroglu, H., Versluis, A., Hellebrekers, L.J., Haberham, Z.L., van Zutphen, L.F.M. and van Lith, H.A. (2003) Strain differences in response to propofol, ketamine and medetomidine in rabbits. *Veterinary Record*, 152:300.

Bateman, L., Ludders, J.W. and Gleed, R.D. (2003) Use of a laryngeal mask airway in rabbits during isoflurane anesthesia. In: *Proceedings of the American College of Veterinary Anesthesiologists, 27th Ann. Meet.*, p. 117, 10–11 October 2002, Orlando.

Cruz, M.I., Sacchi, T., Braz, S.L.J. and Cassu, R. (2000) Use of a laryngeal mask for airway maintenance during inhalation anaesthesia in rabbits. *Veterinary Anaesthesia and Analgesia* 27(2):112–116.

Flecknell, P. (1991) Anaesthesia and post-operative care of small mammals. *Journal of Veterinary Postgraduate Clinical Study in Practice* 13:180–189.

Flecknall, P.A. (1998) Analgesia in small mammals. In: *Seminars in Avian and Exotic Pet Medicine* 7(1):41–47.

Flecknall, P.A. (2000) Anaesthesia. In: *Manual of Rabbit Medicine and Surgery*, 1st edn (ed., Flecknall, P.A.), BSAVA, Cheltenham: 103–116.

Flecknall, P.A. (2006) Anaesthesia and post-operative care. In: *Manual of Rabbit Medicine and Surgery*, 2nd edn (eds, Meredith, A. and Flecknall, P.A.), BSAVA, Quedgeley, Gloucestershire, pp. 154–165.

Girling, S.J. (2003) Small mammal handling and chemical restraint. In: *Veterinary Nursing of Exotic Pets*, Blackwell Publishing, Oxford, pp. 233–245.

Gonzalez Gil, A., Silvan, G., Martinez-Mateos, M.M. and Illera, J.C. (2005) Serum catecholamine levels after halothane and isoflurane anaesthesia in rabbits. *Veterinary Record* 157:589–590.

Hedenqvist, P., Orr, H.E., Roughan, J.V., Antunes, L.M. and Flecknell, P. (2002) Anaesthesia with ketamine medetomidine in the rabbit: influence of the route of administration and the effect of combination with butorphanol. *Veterinary Anaesthesia and Analgesia* 29:14–19.

Malley, D. (2007) Safe handling and restraint of pet rabbits. *In Practice* 29:378–386.

Mason, D.E. (1997) Anesthesia, analgesia and sedation for small mammals. In: *Ferrets, Rabbits and Rodents: Clinical Medicine and Surgery*, 1st edn (eds, Hillyer, E.V. and Quesenberry, K.E.), WB Saunders, Philadelphia, pp. 378–391.

Scheller, M.S., Daidman, L.J. and Partridge, B.L. (1988) MAC of sevoflurane in humans and the New Zealand white rabbit. *Canadian Journal of Anesthesiology* 35:153–156.

# Diagnostic Imaging

# 7.1 Radiography

## 7.1.1 Positioning – general

Poor or incorrect positioning according to Williams (2002) is the commonest reason for non-diagnostic radiographs. To avoid this it is preferable to ensure that the rabbit is immobilised chemically when performing radiography. Two views at 90° to each other are usual: a lateral (usually right) and ventrodorsal or dorsoventral view. In addition, oblique views may be useful when imaging the head, where right and left dental arcades may need to be viewed separately. Rostrocaudal views of the head can also be used to examine the frontal sinuses or temporomandibular joint.

Further information on positioning for specific disease investigation is given in the relevant sections of this chapter.

## 7.1.2 Radiography equipment

*Radiography machine*

The use of a radiographic unit capable of a range of voltages from 40 to 70 kV, with a rapid exposure time of 0.008–0.16 seconds is advised as rabbit respiration rates are rapid and can lead to film blurring (Silverman, 1993). Reduction of the film-focal distance is also a useful feature if possible as this will allow magnification of the image, which can be helpful in smaller rabbits.

Dental radiography machines are also useful to image fine bone structures such as the head and digits, and if combined with non-screen dental film they can provide superior imaging to standard veterinary radiography.

### Grids, film and cassettes

Grids are rarely necessary in the majority of rabbits, due to their smaller size (<10 cm depth of body) (Stefanacci and Hoefer, 2004).

Non-screen dental film, such as the Kodak® series (DF50 and DF75), is extremely useful for dental and distal limb imaging as mentioned above (Girling, 2002). Non-screen mammography film can also be used to enhance soft tissue detail.

Newer cassettes that utilise rare earth phosphors to enhance images are also advised as for other small animals. They allow production of clearer images with lower radiation doses.

## 7.1.3 Interpretation of rabbit radiographs

### Head and associated structures

In the wild European rabbit the head is relatively elongated and slightly flattened from side to side. However, in many domestic breeds (e.g. mini lops and dwarf Netherland) the head has become foreshortened, making it difficult to determine normal anatomy from pathology. The upper jaw contains six 'cheek teeth' (three premolars and three molars) on either side, and the lower jaw contains five cheek teeth (two premolars and three molars) on either side. In the shorter headed domestic breeds, in many cases only five maxillary cheek teeth are seen either side. Inherited mandibular prognathism is also common in the domestic rabbit (Huang et al., 1981) as is brachycephalism (Crossley, 1995).

Rabbits have a dental gap or diastema where the canines would be in cats or dogs. There are four incisors in the upper jaw (maxilla) and two in the lower (mandible) in total. The incisors of the maxilla are arranged so that the accessory incisors or peg teeth are positioned immediately behind the main clearly visible maxillary incisors. The mandibular incisors should then sit in the groove created between these peg teeth and the main maxillary incisors.

It is also worth noting that there should always be a clear gap between the occlusal surfaces of the maxillary and mandibular cheek teeth in the healthy rabbit lateral head radiograph. When overgrowth occurs this is often lost.

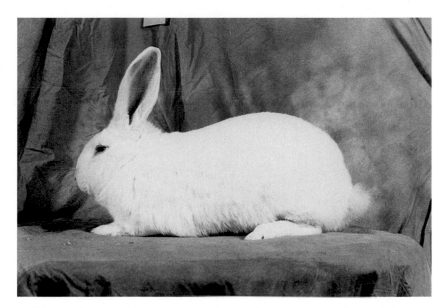

**Colour Plate 1**  British giant. Reproduced with permission from *Fur and Feather* magazine.

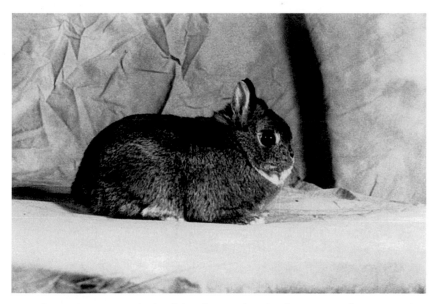

**Colour Plate 2**  Netherland dwarf. Reproduced with permission from *Fur and Feather* magazine.

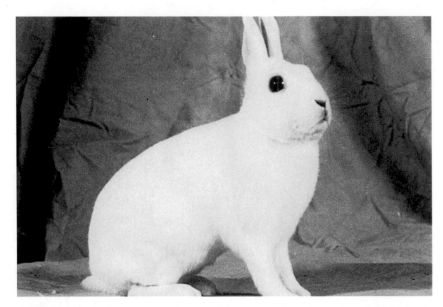

**Colour Plate 3**  Polish. Reproduced with permission from *Fur and Feather* magazine.

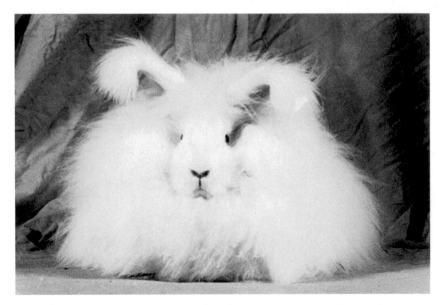

**Colour Plate 4**  Angora. Reproduced with permission from *Fur and Feather* magazine.

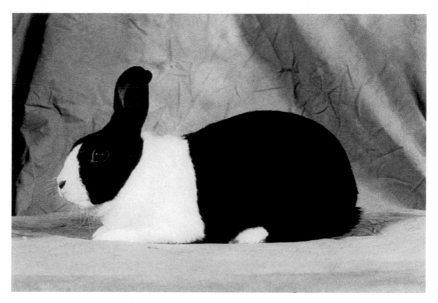

**Colour Plate 5** Dutch. Reproduced with permission from *Fur and Feather* magazine.

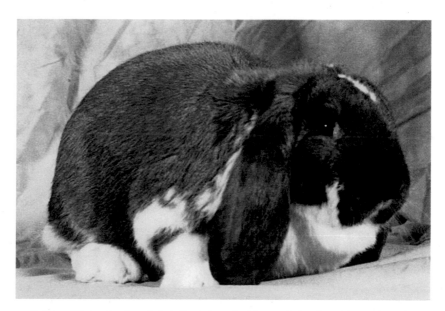

**Colour Plate 6** French lop. Reproduced with permission from *Fur and Feather* magazine.

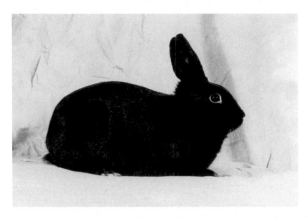

**Colour Plate 7** Havana. Reproduced with permission from *Fur and Feather* magazine.

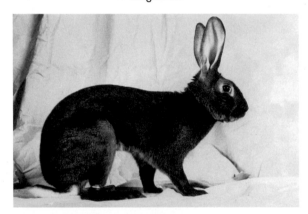

**Colour Plate 8** Belgian hare. Reproduced with permission from *Fur and Feather* magazine.

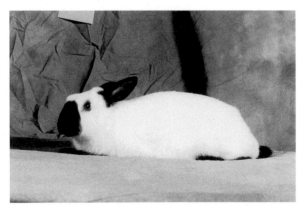

**Colour Plate 9** Himalayan rabbit showing seal point markings. Reproduced with permission from *Fur and Feather* magazine.

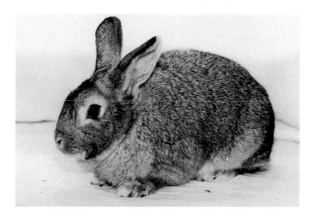

**Colour Plate 10**  Chinchilla. Reproduced with permission from *Fur and Feather* magazine.

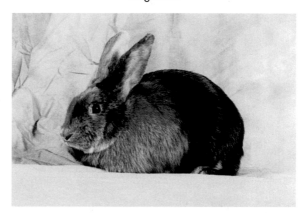

**Colour Plate 11**  Harlequin. Reproduced with permission from *Fur and Feather* magazine.

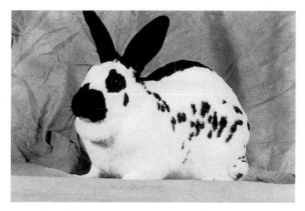

**Colour Plate 12**  English. Reproduced with permission from *Fur and Feather* magazine.

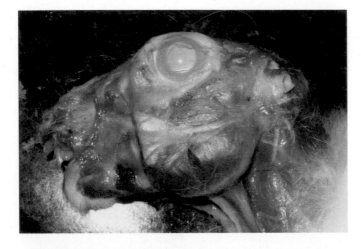

**Colour Plate 13**   Lateral view of rabbit head and neck with the skin removed. Note: Prominent eye and third eyelid; extensive masseter muscles; and the linguofacial vein and retromandibular vein draining the head, which combine further caudally in the neck to create the external jugular vein.

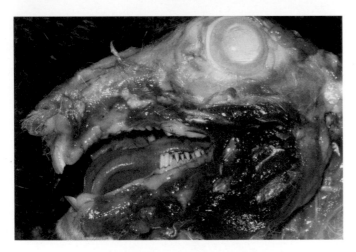

**Colour Plate 14**   Lateral view of rabbit head in Colour Plate 13 with the masseter muscles and lateral cheek removed. Note: Diastema; small peg teeth immediately caudal to the maxillary incisors; fleshy tongue; maxillary and mandibular premolars and molars (so-called cheek teeth).

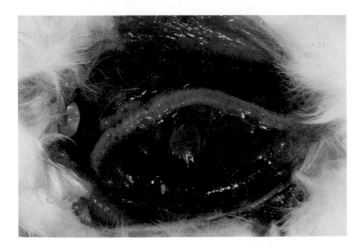

**Colour Plate 15**   Ventral laparotomy approach to the abdomen. The first organs encountered are the extensive caecum and part of the large intestines.

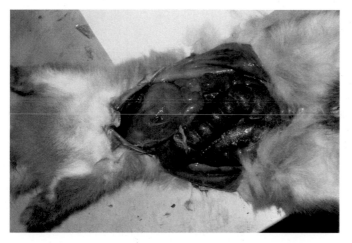

**Colour Plate 16** Post-mortem of a rabbit showing the extensive caecum and large intestines (dark brown) lighter yellow-coloured small intestines (abnormally filled with gas here) and the cream–pink-coloured stomach (which again is abnormally overfilled here).

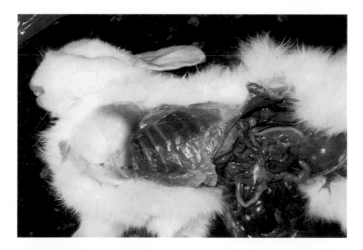

**Colour Plate 17** Lateral view of a rabbit post-mortem with the caecum and large intestines partially reflected ventrally exposing the small intestines. A full urinary bladder can be seen caudally; the stomach may be seen just protruding from behind the ribcage. Note the small size of the thoracic cavity in relation to the abdominal cavity.

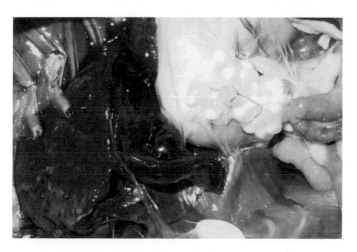

**Colour Plate 18** Close-up from left to right: lungs covering the darker red heart; diaphragm; liver containing the black-coloured gall bladder; cream-coloured stomach. Note the white small fluid-filled structures covering the stomach, which are abnormal and represent the intermediate stage (i.e. *Cysticercus pisiformis*) of the dog and fox tapeworm *Taenia pisiformis*.

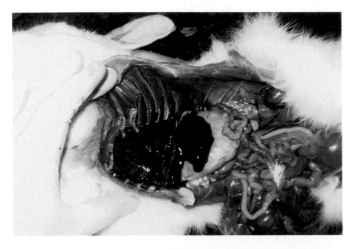

**Colour Plate 19** Lateral post-mortem view of a rabbit with the chest and abdominal walls removed. The structures from left to right (cranial to caudal) are the dark red heart; bright red lungs; darker brown diaphragm and liver; pale cream stomach; yellow brown small intestines (the dark brown large intestines and caecum are reflected ventrally); yellow-coloured urinary bladder. The left kidney may be seen dorsally as a dark brown structure in the mid-abdomen.

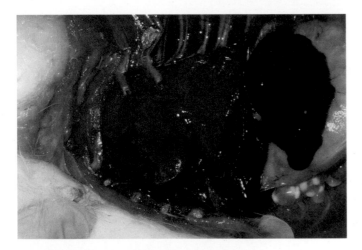

**Colour Plate 20** Close-up of the chest cavity with the lateral wall/ribcage removed. The heart is most cranially situated and overlain by the cranial and middle lobes of the lungs. The thin sheet of diaphragm can be seen separating the lungs from the dark brown liver, which overlies the stomach. Again the abnormal *Cysticercus pisiformis* tapeworm cysts can be seen below the stomach.

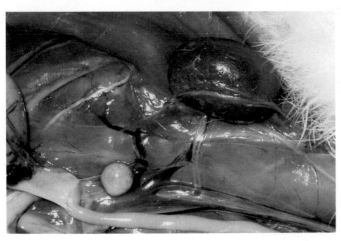

**Colour Plate 21** Close-up of the left kidney showing its venous and arterial connections with the caudal vena cava and aorta, respectively, as well as the ureter, which causes to the bottom right of the picture. Note the white spherical object at bottom left, which is an enlarged left adrenal gland.

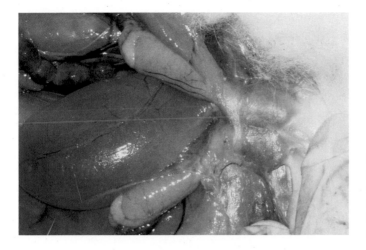

**Colour Plate 22**  Close-up of the caudal abdomen of a male rabbit, showing the retracted testes and the inguinal canals and the full urinary bladder.

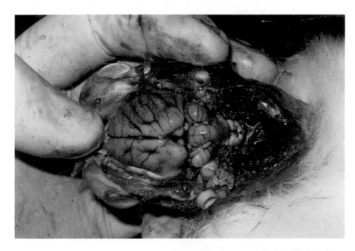

**Colour Plate 23**  Close-up of the cerebrum and cerebellum of the rabbit and their close relation to the external and middle ears.

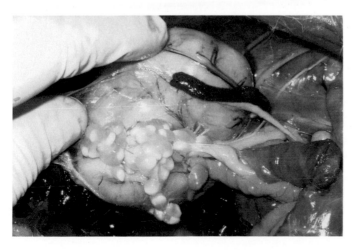

**Colour Plate 24**  Cysts containing tapeworm scolices.

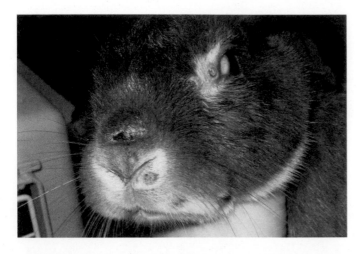

**Colour Plate 25**
Myxomatosis showing crusting around the nose and eyes.

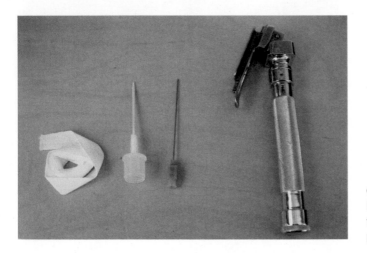

**Colour Plate 26**
Equipment required for tracheostomy. (Originally published in *Vet Times*.)

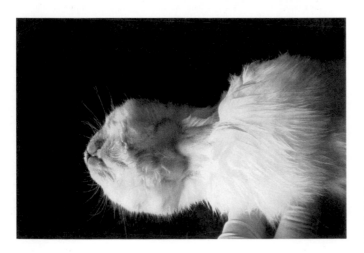

**Colour Plate 27**
Preparation of the tracheostomy site. (Originally published in *Vet Times*.)

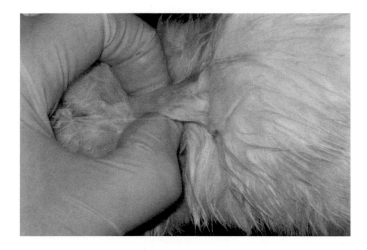

**Colour Plate 28** Grasping the trachea at the site of insertion. (Originally published in *Vet Times*.)

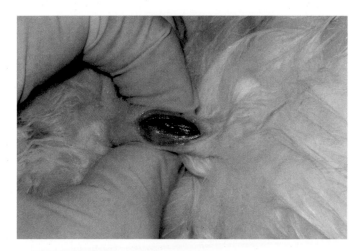

**Colour Plate 29** Initial incision. (Originally published in *Vet Times*.)

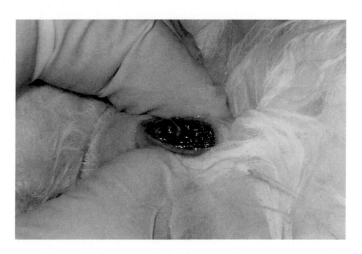

**Colour Plate 30** Tracheal rings are now visible. (Originally published in *Vet Times*.)

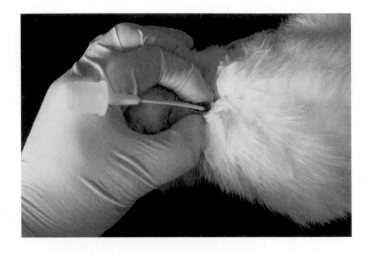

**Colour Plate 31** Insertion of transtracheal catheter. (Originally published in *Vet Times*.)

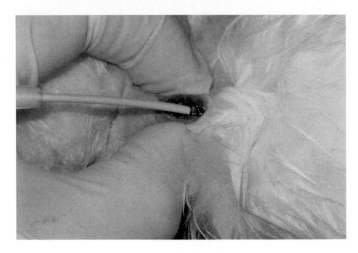

**Colour Plate 32** Closer view of insertion. (Originally published in *Vet Times*.)

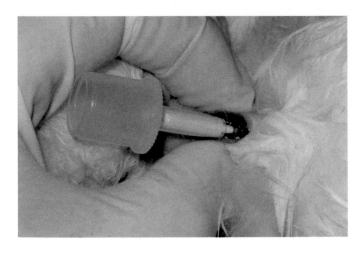

**Colour Plate 33** Final placement of transtracheal catheter. (Originally published in *Vet Times*.)

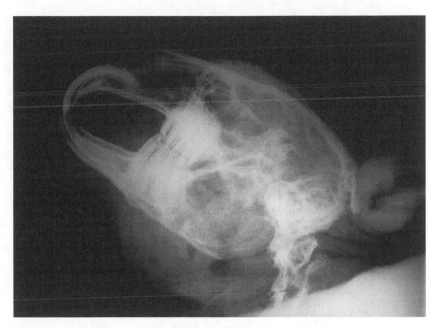

**Figure 7.1** Lateral head showing cheek tooth and incisor malocclusion. Note contact of occlusal surfaces of cheek teeth. Roots of cheek teeth projecting through ventral mandible and upper/lower incisors meeting end on.

Investigation of dental disease in rabbits requires, amongst other things, a radiographic assessment (Harrenstein, 1999). Root elongation, periodontal disease and new bone production as a result of abscessation can often be seen (Fig. 7.1). In the early stages of dental disease, lysis of the alveolar bone is often an early radiographic sign (Redrobe, 2001). As mentioned, cheek teeth may touch each other at rest and this may progress to form a more irregular wave mouth as seen in horses. Irregular wearing of the teeth and changes in their angle of eruption may also be seen. In order that individual root/tooth problems may be examined, oblique views of the skull may be needed to highlight one jaw problem from the opposite side.

Intraoral views using small non-screen film can also be helpful in diagnosing nasal disease, maxillary tooth root problems and ocular disease.

Milky tears due to an oculonasal discharge from a tear duct infection (dacrocystitis), which is usually associated with incisor root elongation or infection as it pinches on the nasolacrimal duct. Contrast studies of the tear ducts may be performed using iodine-based contrast media injected through a cannula into the ventral (and only) punctum (Fig. 7.2).

Middle ear disease is common in rabbits and may result in vestibular disease or torticollis. In these cases a dorsoventral view of the skull

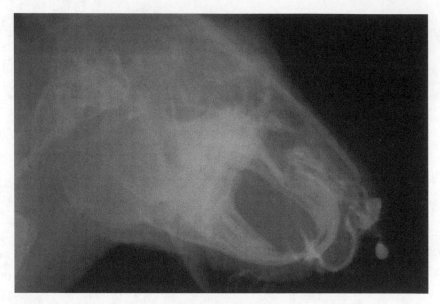

**Figure 7.2** Contrast study of nasolacrimal duct. Note narrowing of duct around root of maxillary incisors.

should be taken to image the bony middle ear. Loss of the fine trabecular structure of the bone with thickening of its walls may be seen with otitis media. A perfectly square on view must be obtained for accuracy (Fig. 7.3).

Tumours of the skull have also been reported in the rabbit such as an osteogenic sarcoma of the mandible (Weisbroth and Hurwitz, 1969), and again oblique views of the mandible may be needed to prevent superimposition with the contralateral jaw.

### Limbs

Of the total body weight of the domestic rabbit on average only 7–8% is made up of skeleton, compared with 12–13% in domestic cats. This leads rabbit bones to be more brittle and this is reflected in the type of fractures seen with comminuted limb fractures being more common in the rabbit. Standard views at 90° (lateral and anterior-posterior/cranial-lateral views) are required.

The skeletal structure of the rabbit differs from the cat in many ways, and some have been mentioned in Chapter 2 and include the posses-sion of clavicles; the presence of a relatively large hooked suprahamate process of the acromion; a triangular infraspinous fossa; small hip joints with large foramina obturata of the pelvis.

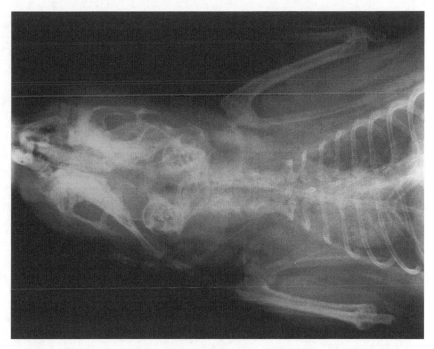

**Figure 7.3** Dorsoventral view showing middle ear disease (worse in right middle ear), dental disease (flaring laterally of first cheek teeth) and enlarged heart.

Luxation of the elbow joint or hip has been reported. In addition, septic arthritis of the phalangeal or tarsal joints due to pododermatitis is commonly seen. In older rabbits as with other animals, osteoarthritis is another regularly seen feature of limb radiographs.

Neoplasia, such as fibrosarcomas and osteosarcomas, are also not uncommon in rabbits, with fibrosarcomas often affecting distal limbs and osteosarcomas commonly affecting the humerus, femur and tibia. Hypertrophic osteopathy associated with an intrathoracic neoplasm (DeSanto, 1997) and a limb neurofibrosarcoma in association with a thymic neoplasm (Clippinger *et al.*, 1998) have also been recorded.

### Spine and ribs

The rabbit spine is long in proportion to its overall size and generally held curved at rest. The normal vertebral formula is for seven cervical vertebrae, twelve thoracic, seven lumbar, four sacral and approximately sixteen coccygeal vertebrae. Some individuals do possess thirteen thoracic vertebrae (Kozma *et al.*, 1974). Vertebral fractures and sub/luxations of the spine are common in rabbits, particularly so in individuals suffering from osteoporotic conditions due to metabolic bone disease. Vertebral fractures may be compression or complex in type and young rabbits may show vertebral growth plate fractures. Positioning is as for other small animals with a standard right lateral and a dorsoventral view of the spine being preferred.

Spondylosis lesions have been recorded in the rabbit (Green *et al.*, 1984). These could affect rabbits as young as 3 months of age in some cases, although most rabbits were 2 or more years old. Myelography may be used to assess disc rupture as a result of trauma or spondylosis. The L6/7 intervertebral space is used for introduction of 0.4 mL/kg of an iodine contrast medium (Longley, 2005).

The ribs are attached to the sternum, with the exception of pairs 8 and 9 which are fused to the seventh pair and ribs 10–12 which are not attached to the rest, but end freely in the abdominal wall muscles.

## Thorax

Two views, a traditional right lateral and a dorsoventral view, are generally preferred (Figs 7.4 and 7.5). Care should be taken to draw the forelimbs well forward so as to avoid obstructing the cardiac shadow and precardiac/thymus area.

The heart seems abnormally large on normal rabbit radiographs as the chest cavity in rabbits is small in comparison to their overall body

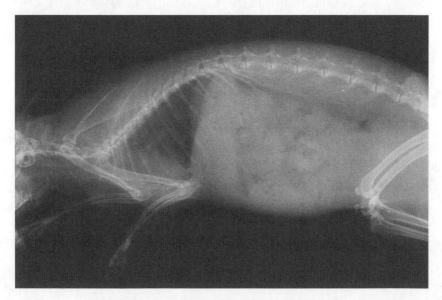

**Figure 7.4** Lateral view of normal rabbit.

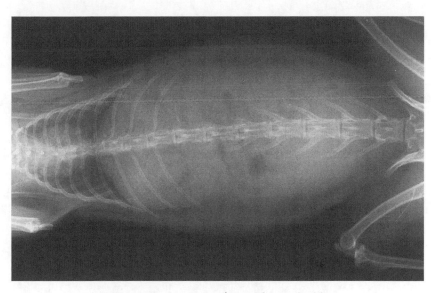

**Figure 7.5** Dorsoventral view of normal rabbit.

size. The heart occupies most of the cranioventral part of the chest, i.e. the fourth to sixth rib spaces. Fat deposits are common in overweight rabbits around the heart itself and can further increase the cardiac outline. However, true cardiac enlargement due to disease is common in the rabbit and maybe due to valvular disease or cardiomyopathy. Other cardiovascular abnormalities that may be seen include an increased density of the main blood vessels entering and exiting the heart in cases of atherosclerosis in obese rabbits (Shell and Saunders, 1989) or where dietary over-supplementation of calcium and vitamin D3 has occurred, leading to calcification of the wall of the vessels.

The thymus lies cranial to the heart and can be seen on lateral radiographs even in the adult rabbit. Neoplasia (both adenoma and lymphoma) of the thymus has been recorded and may lead to the heart shadow being pushed caudally in addition to creating a precardiac shadow.

The actual overall lung size of rabbits in relation to body mass is small, which makes identifying lung disease difficult. Consolidation of one or more lung lobes due to chronic infection or abscesses may be seen, but air alveolograms and air bronchograms are more difficult to observe in rabbits as a consequence. Other more obvious conditions include certain neoplasms, e.g. uterine adenocarcinomas that metastasise to the lungs. Lateral views of the chest are preferable in the rabbit to detect these lesions, although a dorsoventral view is still necessary to pinpoint which lung the lesion resides in.

Pleural effusions may also be seen in rabbits, as with cats with a space occupying density in between the chest wall and outer lung surface, as well as widening the mediastinal space.

### Abdomen

Positioning of the rabbit for imaging most of the abdominal organs requires two views: a lateral and a ventrodorsal or dorsoventral. It may be helpful to perform a right and left lateral view in some cases where obstructions are suspected. The hindlimbs should be pulled caudally in both lateral and ventrodorsal/dorsoventral views to prevent their overlying the area being imaged.

### Intestines

In contrast to the thoracic cavity, the abdominal cavity appears relatively large in the rabbit. The predominant organs are the large intestines and caecum. The caecum is found on the right side of the abdomen and ventrally. In the healthy rabbit the caecum should be full of semifluid ingesta with a few small gas bubbles. Excessive build-up of gas can occur in cases of bloat associated with colic and gut stasis, which is seen in cases of mucoid enteropathy (Fig. 7.6). The descending colon and rectum in the healthy rabbit contains faecal pellets.

### Stomach

The stomach should always contain ingesta in healthy rabbits. Excessive gas in the stomach (Figs 7.7 and 7.8) may again indicate gut stasis, although small volumes may be normal. The stomach should not normally extend beyond the caudal rib margin, but fur and ingesta matted material (so-called trichobezoars) may result in this. To help outline the contents of the stomach to determine if a trichobezoar is present, barium sulphate positive contrast media may be administered at 10–15 mL/kg by nasogastric or orogastric tube. Gastric emptying and intestinal motility are difficult to assess in the rabbit as the stomach is always full and some liquid barium, if used, will remain in the stomach for several days. One such contrast study indicated that 32% of a liquid marker reaches the caecum in 1 hour and 80% by 12 hours in the healthy rabbit (Pickard and Stevens, 1972), whereas solid markers (radiodense beads) reached the caecum within 4 hours.

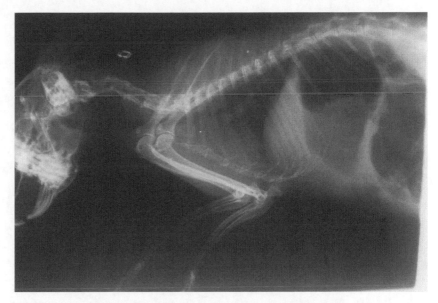

**Figure 7.6** Gastric and intestinal bloat as a result of penicillin toxicity. Chest cavity is normal. The radiodense object over the neck is a staple in a skin wound.

### Liver

The liver is much more flattened from cranial to caudal in the rabbit than in cats and dogs. It is normally situated completely underneath the caudal ribcage and cranial to the stomach. Cases of fatty liver degeneration (hepatic lipidosis), hepatic coccidiosis (due to *Eimeria stiediae* infections) and liver abscessation may enlarge the liver shadow and push the stomach outline more caudally and dorsally.

### Kidneys

The renal shadows of the rabbit are similar to that seen in the cat. Each renal shadow should average 1.4–2.2 times the length of the second lumbar vertebra with a mean of 1.8 times in the healthy rabbit (Girling, 2006). Abnormalities include renal and ureteral stones/calculi which are usually very radiodense (and also very painful for the rabbit) as shown in Figures 7.9 and 7.10. Excretory urograms may be useful in assessing renal disease. These are performed using 2 mL/kg of an intravenous iodine-based contrast media injected into a peripheral vein and then quickly radiographing the rabbit to show the movement of the contrast

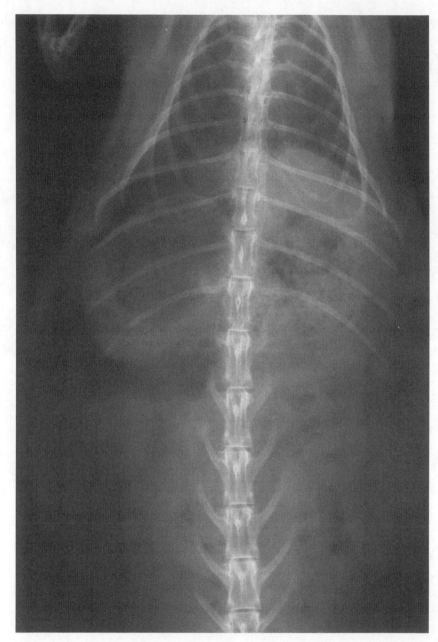

**Figure 7.7** Dorsoventral radiograph of gastric dilatation associated with a foreign body. Note stomach projecting behind rib cage.

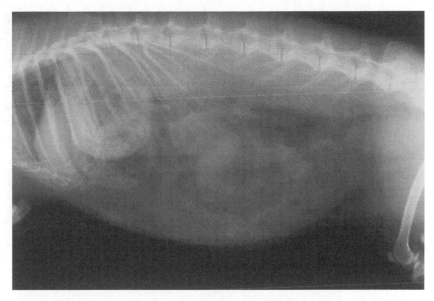

**Figure 7.8**  Lateral view of Figure 7.7 showing dilated stomach and gas loops in small intestine.

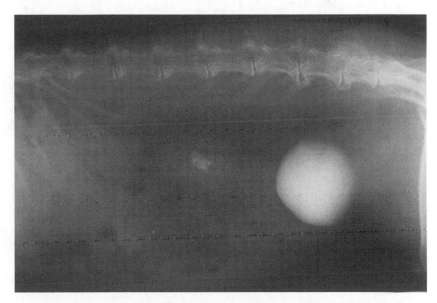

**Figure 7.9**  Lateral abdomen showing radiodense calculi in left kidney and radiodense silt in bladder. Note spondylosis lesions in L5–6 and L6–7.

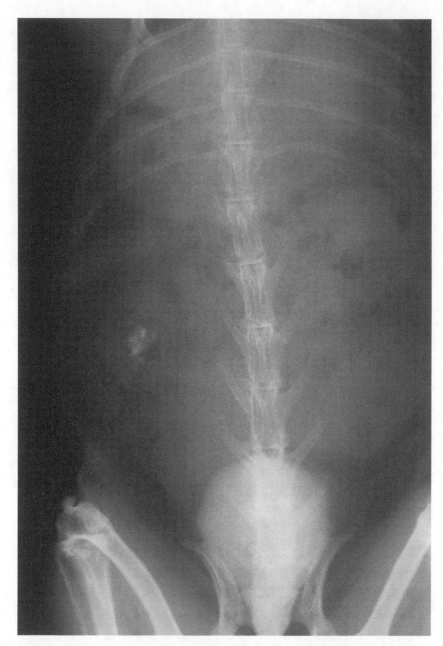

**Figure 7.10**   Dorsoventral view of rabbit in Figure 7.9 showing multiple radiodense calculi in left kidney and radiodense silt in urinary bladder.

media through the circulation to the kidneys where it should be excreted uniformly from both kidneys.

### Urinary bladder

Even in normal, apparently healthy, rabbits, the bladder is often highlighted by the presence of calcium carbonate crystals which commonly form in their urine. Excessive amounts of the silt-like material may block the bladder and create an intense shadow outline of the viscus. Larger solitary calculi may also be seen. The urinary bladder lining can be imaged by using negative contrast techniques with air at 5–8 mL/kg body weight injected into the bladder via a urethral 3–3.5 French Teflon®–coated urinary catheter. In addition, as with dogs and cats, double contrast techniques may then be employed by injecting an iodine-based contrast media at a rate of 2–3 mL/kg.

### Uterus

An enlarged uterus can occur due to neoplasia (e.g. uterine adenocarcinomas), pyometra or gravidity. Venous aneurysms have also been recorded in the vagina of certain rabbit breeds (New Zealand whites) and may also be responsible for causing reproductive tract enlargement in the doe.

### Male reproductive system

The testes can be retracted into the caudal abdomen along with their fat pads and may occasionally confuse the clinician by masquerading as abdominal masses. The penis of male rabbits has no bone/*os penis* running through it.

### Vascular and other abnormalities

Loss of detail in the abdominal cavity may occur with peritonitis, or often combined with distension of the abdomen may suggest ascites which is common with right-sided heart failure.

Increased radiodensity of the abdominal blood vessels can occur with calcification due to calcium/vitamin D3 imbalances and with atherosclerosis.

## 7.2 Ultrasonography

### 7.2.1 Positioning and preparation

A right lateral position, using a cut-out imaging window in the table below as for cats and dogs, is useful for the examination of the heart and kidneys, but it can be stressful to some patients and may require prior sedation.

A standing position, or where the hindlimbs are in contact with the table but a handler lifts the front limbs into the air, is often better tolerated and allows easier access to the liver and many other abdominal organs.

When preparing the patient for ultrasound examination, it is preferable to shave the fur over the area to be imaged and apply coupling gel several minutes prior to imaging to allow the gel to soak into the skin surface and provide a good contact.

### 7.2.2 Equipment

A sector transducer is preferable to a linear one due to its smaller head/footprint, which is useful when imaging smaller animals. The higher frequencies of probes are also preferable considering the smaller size of the patient; therefore, 5–7.5 MHz are required for most rabbits although 10 MHz probes may be useful for imaging the eye. B mode ultrasound as with cats and dogs is the main mode used for visceral organ imaging. The exception is the use of M mode when imaging the heart to assess chamber emptying and contractility. Doppler techniques for assessing blood flow direction and the measurement of ejection volumes with continuous wave Doppler are also used in rabbits to look for cardiac defects.

Stand-offs may be needed for imaging very small structures such as the eye. These can be commercially made which provide the best quality images, or home made from latex gloves filled with coupling gel. Using a printer or recording device helps compare images from previous examinations as well as gives something to help explain problems to the owner.

### 7.2.3 Interpretation of ultrasound images

*Thorax*

The rabbit heart is similar in construction to the cat or dog with a few differences including the presence of only two atrioventricular valves in the right side as opposed to the three seen in other species.

Ultrasound studies of the heart have been described in the rabbit (Tello de Meneses *et al.*, 1989; Marano *et al.*, 1997; Redrobe, 2001). Many different cardiac conditions have been recorded in rabbits, but the more commonly seen include atrioventricular valve defects/insufficiency and particularly dilated cardiomyopathies (chiefly in older rabbits with atherosclerosis) (Orcutt, 2000). In addition, bacterial endocarditis has been reported (Snyder *et al.*, 1976) and may be diagnosed by ultrasonography as may atherosclerosis and associated thrombi.

Anaesthetics, if used, may affect the heart contractions and be detectable using echocardiography. Isoflurane has less of an effect on reducing myocardial contractility than halothane, for example (Marano *et al.*, 1997). Indeed, Marini and others (1999) used ultrasonography to highlight myocardial fibrosis associated with ketamine/xylazine anaesthesia in rabbits.

The thymus is present even in adult rabbits and may be imaged through the heart.

*Abdomen*

The liver is approached from a ventral aspect just caudal to the caudal edge of the sternum. Liver diseases such as hepatic lipidosis may be diagnosed as an increase in echogenicity. Abscesses in the liver may be seen as hyperechoic structures with a thickened capsule. The gallbladder may also be readily seen.

The kidneys may be imaged from mid-caudal abdomen and due to their mobility and pliable abdominal wall, from the ventral or lateral aspects although using the urinary bladder as an 'acoustic window' can sometime improve the quality of images. The normal kidney structure is bean shaped similar to that seen in the cat, although rabbits are uni-papillate, that is the collecting ducts meet at one papilla which empties into the renal calyx and so into the ureter. Examination of the kidneys may show disruption of the renal papilla, distortion of the medulla and cortex and irregularity of the kidney outline all of which may indicate inflammation or neoplasia. Decrease in renal size may indicate chronic renal failure and if combined with an irregular outline is suggestive of *Encephalitozoon cuniculi* damage.

The urinary bladder, as with other species, can be used as an acoustic window to assess organs such as the uterus and kidneys. However, the common occurrence of calcium carbonate crystals in the urine may cause a 'snow-storm' effect limiting the ultrasound image.

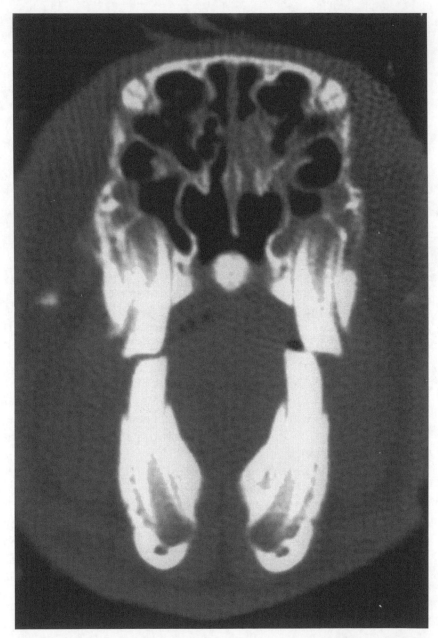

**Figure 7.11** CT scan showing transverse section of rabbit head. Courtesy of Alison King (the Diagnostic Imaging Department, Glasgow University Veterinary School).

The uterus is best imaged from the ventral aspect via the urinary bladder. Abnormalities which may be detected include uterine adenocarcinomas as well as pyometra and venous aneurysms within the vagina. Pregnancy diagnosis may also be performed relatively easily after day 14.

### Eye

As mentioned, a 10 MHz probe is required for this and can be used to determine ocular disease such as lymphoma, ocular abscesses and uveitis lesions caused by lens rupture due to *E. cuniculi*. In addition, diagnosis of retrobulbar masses may be performed (Redrobe, 2001).

## 7.3 MRI and CT scanning

Computed tomography (CT) scanning uses X-rays to create a cross sectional image of the patient (Fig. 7.11). As with radiography it is particularly good for assessing bony changes such as tumours, osteoarthritis and middle ear disease. The patient must be anaesthetised to keep totally still. It is not such a useful modality for assessing soft tissue problems.

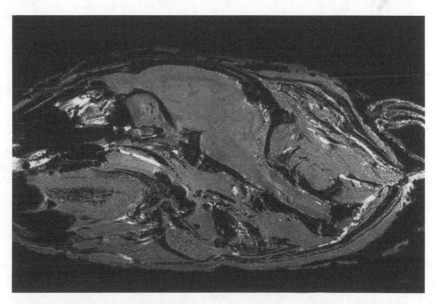

**Figure 7.12** MRI scan of saggital section of rabbit head. Courtesy of Alison King (the Diagnostic Imaging Department, Glasgow University Veterinary School).

Magnetic resonance imaging (MRI) is more useful for assessing soft tissue structures, such as aneurysms, tumours and organ enlargement (Fig. 7.12). It also requires the patient to be anaesthetised and completely immobile. Because MRI can penetrate bone without distorting the image, it is ideal for use in imaging structures such as the brain. In rabbits, spinal abscesses (Runge *et al.*, 1998) and pyelonephritis (Runge *et al.*, 1997) have been assessed using MRI.

# References

Clippinger, T.L., Bennett, R.A., Alleman, A.R., Ginn, P.E. and Bellah, J.R. (1998) Removal of a thymoma via median sternotomy in a rabbit with recurrent appendicular neurofibrosarcoma. *Journal of the American Veterinary Medical Association* 213:1140–1143.

Crossley, D.A. (1995) Clinical aspects of lagomorph dental anatomy: the rabbit (*Oryctolagus cuniculus*). *Journal of Veterinary Dentistry* 12:137–140.

DeSanto, J. (1997) Hypertrophic osteopathy associated with an intrathoracic neoplasm in a rabbit. *Journal of the American Veterinary Medical Association* 210:1322–1323.

Girling, S.J. (2002) Mammalian imaging and anatomy. In: *Manual of Exotic Pets*, 4th edn (eds, Meredith, A. and Redrobe, S.), BSAVA, Quedgeley, pp. 1–12.

Girling, S.J. (2006) Diagnostic imaging. In: *Manual of Rabbits*, 2nd edn (eds, Meredith, A. and Flecknall, P.), BSAVA, Quedgeley, Gloucestershire, pp. 51–62.

Green, P.W., Fox, R.R. and Sokoloff, L. (1984) Spontaneous degenerative spinal disease in the laboratory rabbit. *Journal of Orthopaedic Research* 2:161–168.

Harrenstein, L. (1999) Gastrointestinal diseases of pet rabbits. *Seminars in Avian and Exotic Pet Medicine* 8:83–99.

Huang, C.M., Mi, M.P. and Vogt, D.W. (1981) Mandibular prognathism in the rabbit: discrimination between single-locus and multifactorial models of inheritance. *The Journal of Heredity* 72:296–298.

Kozma, C., Macklin, W., Cummins, L.M. and Mauer, R. (1974) Anatomy, physiology and biochemistry of the rabbit. In: *The Biology of the Laboratory Rabbit*, Academic Press, New York, pp. 50–72.

Longley, L. (2005) Epidural catheterisation in rabbits. In: *Proceedings of the British Veterinary Zoological Society Spring Meeting*, Chester 2005, pp. 56–57.

Marano, G., Formigari, R., Grigioni, M. and Vergari, A. (1997) Effects of isoflurane versus halothane on myocardial contractility in rabbits: assessment with transthoracic two-dimensional echocardiography. *Laboratory Animal Science* 31:144–150.

Marini, R.P., Li, X., Harpster, N.K. and Dangler, C. (1999) Cardiovascular pathology possibly associated with ketamine/xylazine anesthesia in Dutch belted rabbits. *Laboratory Animal Science* 49:153–160.

Orcutt, C.J. (2000) Cardiac and respiratory disease in rabbits. In: *Proceedings of the British Veterinary Zoological Society, Autumn Meeting RVC London*, pp. 68–73.

Pickard, D.W. and Stevens, C.E. (1972) Digesta flow through the rabbit large intestine. *American Journal of Physiology* 222:1161–1166.

Redrobe, S. (2001) Imaging small mammals. *Seminars in Avian and Exotic Pet Medicine* 10:187–197.

Runge, V.M., Timoney, J.F. and Williams, N.M. (1997) Magnetic resonance imaging of experimental pyelonephritis in rabbits. *Investigative Radiology* 32:696–701.

Runge, V.M., Williams, N.M., Lee, C. and Timoney, J.F. (1998) MRI imaging in a spinal abscess model. Preliminary report. *Investigative Radiology* 33:246–255.

Shell, L.G. and Saunders, G. (1989) Arteriosclerosis in a rabbit. *Journal of the American Veterinary Medical Association* 194:679–680.

Silverman, S. (1993) Diagnostic imaging of exotic pets. *Veterinary Clinics of North America: Small Animal Practice* 23:1287–1299.

Snyder, S.B., Fox, J.G., Campbell, L.H. and Soave, O.A. (1976) Disseminated staphylococcal disease in laboratory rabbits (*Oryctolagus cuniculus*). *Laboratory Animal Science* 26:86–88.

Stefanacci, J.D. and Hoefer, H.L. (2004) Radiology and ultrasound. In: *Ferrets, Rabbits and Rodents, Clinical Medicine and Surgery*, 2nd edn (eds, Quesenberry, K.E. and Carpenter, J.W.), WB Saunders, Philadelphia, pp. 395–413.

Tello de Meneses, R., Mesa, M.D. and Gonzalez, V. (1989) Echocardiographic assessment of cardiac function in the rabbit: a preliminary study. *Annales de recherches veterinaires* 20:175–185.

Weisbroth, S.H. and Hurwitz, A. (1969) Spontaneous osteogenic sarcoma in *Oryctolagus cuniculus* with elevated serum alkaline phosphatase. *Laboratory Animal Care* 19:263–265.

Williams, J. (2002) Orthopaedic radiography in exotic animal practice. *Veterinary Clinics of North America: Exotic Animal Practice* 5(1):1–22.

# General Concepts of Nursing

8

## 8.1 Introduction

Before we examine specific conditions of rabbits, we will spend some time looking at the theories of nursing that are currently applied to nursing of cats and dogs and examine how they relate to the nursing of rabbits.

The most important thing when dealing with rabbits is to remember that rabbits are prey species and their behaviour will be affected by the presence of humans. Do not be tempted to dive in and start handling the rabbit without observing it first. Patient observation ideally should take place from outside the kennel room if at all possible. This may allow you to see if the rabbit is eating, drinking or moving about. Once you enter the kennel room, some rabbits will move to the back of the cage and not do anything – so if information can be gathered beforehand, so much the better. Parameters that you should try to record from a distance are listed in Box 8.1.

After examining the patients from a distance, they can be observed more closely but still not handling them. Again the parameters mentioned in Box 8.1 should be recorded.

## 8.2 Basic clinical examination

The basic clinical examination of the rabbit is similar to that of the cat or dog. After observing the rabbit from a distance, it can be observed more closely and then finally handled. Parameters which should be noted are described in Table 8.1.

---

> **Box 8.1 Parameters which should be observed from a distance**
>
> 1. Demeanour – is the rabbit bright or dull?
> 2. Movement – is the rabbit moving round the cage or sitting at the back of the cage?
> 3. Eating – have you observed the rabbit eating?
> 4. Interacting with others – if there is another rabbit in the cage, are they interacting with each other?
> 5. Breathing – does breathing appear laboured?
> 6. Any other problems observed?

## 8.3 Administration of medication

The routes of administration in rabbits are similar to those of cats and dogs – namely oral, subcutaneous, intramuscular (see Fig. 8.1), intraperitoneal, intravenous and intra-osseous. Advantages and disadvantages

**Table 8.1** Parameters to examine and record when carrying out a physical examination

| Parameter | Comment |
|-----------|---------|
| Body condition | Emaciated, thin, normal, overweight. How prominent are the vertebrae? |
| Skin/coat | Are there any areas of alopecia, crusting, sores or scurf? |
| | Make sure to examine the hocks and perineal area |
| Body temperature | Normal |
| Pulse/auscultation | Normal heart rate 180–250 bpm. Can reach 330 bpm in excited rabbit |
| | Use femoral artery as in dog/cat to record pulse |
| | Can any crackles be heard over the lungs? |
| | How easy is it to hear the heart beat? |
| Jugular distension | Can be difficult to see in some breeds due to coat. Suggests venous congestion |
| Respiratory rate | Normal respiratory rate |
| | Is respiration laboured? |
| | Is the rabbit mouth breathing? |
| | Is orthopnoea present? |
| Mucous membrane colour/ capillary refill time Obvious incisor problems | Pink. Capillary refill time of ~2 seconds normal |
| Discharge from the nose Discharge from the eyes | Mucoid, purulent uni/bilateral |
| Ears | Crusting |

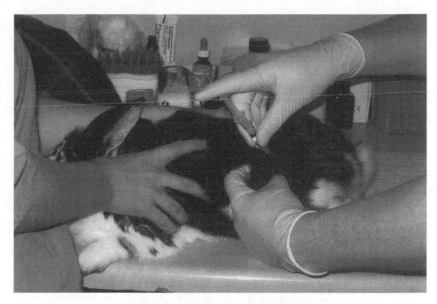

**Figure 8.1**  Intramuscular injection.

of each relate to the degree of hydration and blood supply. Choice of route depends on the medication being given, the speed of effect that is wanted and the area of the body being treated.

## 8.4 Nursing models

Nursing models have been used for many years within the field of human nursing and are now being applied to the veterinary nursing profession. The basic nursing model consists of four stages: assessment, planning, implementation (or intervention) and evaluation. We now look at each of these stages in turn.

### 8.4.1 Assessment

The assessment stage involves obtaining the animal's history and the clinical examination. Examples of the type of information that need to be collected during this stage are given in Table 8.2.

### 8.4.2 Planning

In this stage you will decide what nursing care is needed for the patients based on your assessment of their needs. Examples of the points noted

**Table 8.2** Information that should be gathered for the assessment stage

| Information | Examples |
|---|---|
| Why is the animal being hospitalised? | Elective surgery<br>Assisted feeding |
| How old is the animal? | Young, middle aged, old |
| Will the rabbit have a 'cage buddy'? | Other rabbit |
| Has the owner provided any bedding? | Newspaper, straw, etc. |
| How long will the rabbit be in the hospital? | Less than a day or long term |
| How is the rabbit normally provided with water? | Bottle or bowl |
| What is the rabbit normally fed? | Type of fruit or vegetables the rabbit likes |
| What type of accommodation will the patient need? | Small kennel or large kennel to accommodate kennel mate |
| What type of assistance will the patient need? | Assisted feeding |
| Body temperature | Is this normal, pyrexic, below normal? |
| How often should the animal be fed? | — |
| Is medication required? | How often should this be given? |
| Does the rabbit require exercise? | How often should this be given? |
| Is the rabbit in pain? | Provision of analgesia |

during the planning stage are given in Box 8.2. The nursing plan also needs to include contingency planning for things going wrong, such as the animal developing other problems, not responding to treatment, or developing side-effects from the current treatment. Therefore, you can see that the nursing plan is not a fixed thing – it will change from day to day or even hour to hour. It is also important that the nursing plan fits in with the way in which the veterinary surgeon wishes to treat the animal.

---

**Box 8.2 Examples of some points noted during the planning stage**

1. What will the rabbit be fed?
2. How often will they be fed?
3. How much food will be given?
4. How often will the amount of food eaten be monitored?
5. How often will fresh food be given?
6. What type of accommodation will the rabbit be given?
7. What medication is required?
8. How often will this be given?
9. How often will exercise be allowed?
10. What type of analgesia should be given?

Communication between both the veterinary nurse and the veterinary surgeon is vital.

### 8.4.3 Implementation

As the name suggests, this is when you actually nurse the patient.

### 8.4.4 Evaluation

This is the stage when you examine the outcome of your nursing care. Hopefully, this is when the patient gets better, but it is possible that the patient could deteriorate or develop other conditions.

The way in which this plan is laid out can suggest that this is a long process. However, in reality the nursing plan is something that all nurses will already be carrying out – just not in this formal manner. Evaluation will take place at the same time as implementation and will also take place on a daily basis when ward rounds are being carried out or when there is a change of staff. Using a nursing model such as this can be helpful to ensure that all points are noted down, and that all information is recorded when more than one member of staff is dealing with a patient.

An example of a nursing model for a rabbit patient is given in Table 8.3.

Various versions of this nursing model have been used in human nursing. The two versions which are now being in veterinary nursing are the Roper, Logan and Tierney model and the Orem model.

### 8.4.5 Roper, Logan and Tierney model

The basis of this model (Roper et al. (1996)) is to relate the nursing care of the patient to the normal activities of daily living. The authors described 12 activities of human daily living which they considered normal. These include things such as breathing, eating, moving about, sleeping and keeping clean.

### 8.4.6 Orem model

Orem's model (1991) also follows the basic concepts of assessment, planning, implementation and evaluation, but it focuses the nursing care on the ability of the patient to care for themselves. The role of the veterinary nursing therefore is to make up the deficit between what the

**Table 8.3** Nursing plan for a 1-year-old Angora rabbit with dental disease

| Parameter | Comment |
|---|---|
| Assessment | |
| Why is the animal being hospitalised? | Dental surgery. Animal is currently anorexic. Has not been eating for 24 hours |
| Age of animal | Young |
| temperature, pulse, respiration | Normal |
| Food required | Normally would eat a variety of food, but has been admitted for dental treatment. May not be willing to eat |
| Water | Normally given via a bottle |
| Accommodation | Is the rabbit a house rabbit or an outdoor rabbit? Does the rabbit use a litter tray? What type of litter is the rabbit used to? |
| Analgesia | Will be required |
| Medication | Will be required |
| Grooming | Long-coated breed with dental disease – may be matted |
| Any other possible problems? | Gut stasis if not eating |
| Planning | |
| Type of kennel for the rabbit | In exotics ward. Warm (20°C). Provision of hay and bolt-hole. Provision of litter tray |
| Food | Fresh food always available. Pieces of fresh vegetable to be counted in and out to record amount eaten. If not eating then assisted feeding required |
| Grooming | Groom whilst anaesthetised and then daily whilst hospitalised |
| Medication | |
| Analgesia | |
| Provision of exercise | Allow to exercise twice daily for 30 minutes after day of surgery |
| Preoperative requirements | |
| Postoperative requirements | |
| Implementation | Anything observed at the time of nursing? |
| Evaluation | How successful was the nursing care given? What needs to be changed? |

animals should do to care for themselves and what they are able to do. For example, if the patient is not able to groom himself or herself, then the veterinary nurse will need to carry this out. Orem listed eight self-care requisites for humans, which can also be applied to animals (see Box 8.3). If using this model then you would think about these parameters and how you could assist the animal. So for example, in the case of a rabbit with faecal matting and flystrike, keeping the rabbit clean would allow it to defaecate normally. Keeping the rabbit in accommodation, which is away from prey animals such as cats, would be a prevention of hazards.

---

**Box 8.3   Orem's self-care requisite**

1. Provision of air
2. Provision of water
3. Provision of food
4. Elimination of waste
5. A balance between activity and rest
6. A balance between solitude and social interaction
7. Prevention of hazards
8. To feel normal in relation to others

---

### 8.4.7 Home care

The nursing models described have concentrated on the care of the rabbit whilst in the veterinary practice. However, many patients will require some form of care at home. Many practices are now providing owners with care sheets at the time of discharge. For rabbits, it is important that owners are aware of just how important it is that their pets continue to eat. It is not unusual for a rabbit to be seen eating in the practice and then become anorexic when sent home. If owners are not aware of just how serious gut stasis can be then the rabbit can become very ill or even die. The basic concepts of nursing care – assessment, planning, implementing and evaluating – can be designed for the owners. The vet and/or the veterinary nurse can have input to the assessment of the patient and the planning of the home care. This can be discussed with the owner at a discharge appointment and written instructions given to the owner. The evaluation of this care can then take place at the follow-up appointment with either the vet or the veterinary nursing depending on the individual condition. Evaluation can also take place over the phone – a follow-up call the day after discharge will allow the owner to ask any questions and ensure that they are following the instructions. Any problems can be identified early on.

## 8.5 Specific procedures

### 8.5.1 Blood sampling

Venous access has already been described in Chapter 6. The most commonly used vessel for venous access is the lateral ear vein, but it is

**Table 8.4** Normal plasma/serum biochemical parameters and urinalysis results for healthy adult rabbits (see also Table 2.3 pg 25 of Haenatological values for rabbits)

| Parameter | Value in a healthy domestic rabbit |
|---|---|
| Urine volume | 10–35 mL/kg/day average (depending on diet) |
| Urine specific gravity | 1.003–1.036 |
| Urine erythrocyte numbers | <5 erythrocytes per high power field |
| Urine protein levels | Trace to absent (may be more in juveniles) |
| Urine colour | Varies from pale yellow to deep red, depending on presence/absence of porphyrins |
| Urine average pH | 8.2 |
| Urine crystals | Small volumes of ammonium magnesium phosphate or calcium carbonate are normal |
| Plasma proteins | 44–82 g/L |
| Serum albumin | 24–59 g/L (54.4% average of TP) |
| Serum alpha globulins | Average 11.6% of TP (often split alpha-1 and -2 peaks) |
| Serum beta-1 globulins | Average 11.9% of TP |
| Serum beta-2 globulins | Average 5.8% of TP |
| Serum gamma globulins | Average 11.2% of TP |
| Albumin/globulin ratio | Average 1.64 |
| Plasma urea | 2.9–17.1 mmol/L |
| Plasma creatinine | 44–248 umol/L |
| Endogenous creatine clearance rate | 2.2–4.2 mL/minute/kg |
| Plasma phosphorus | 1.42–2.33 mmol/L |
| Plasma potassium | 2.2–6.2 mmol/L |
| Plasma sodium | 135–161 mmol/L |
| Plasma calcium | 2–3.88 mmol/L |
| Ionised plasma calcium | Average 1.71 mmol/L |
| Packed cell volume | 30–50% |
| Red blood cell count | $4–8 \times 10^{12}$/L |

possible to use the cephalic, saphenous or jugular veins. Normal values for haematology and biochemistry can be found in Tables 8.4 and 8.5.

## 8.5.2 Blood pressure monitoring/using a pulse oximeter

Blood pressure monitoring is now more common in cats and dogs and is something that can be used in rabbits. Traditionally, blood pressure is recorded as a systolic value (when the heart contracts) and a diastolic value (when the heart relaxes). See Table 8.6 for more information.

The forelimb can be used in rabbits to obtain a blood pressure measurement. The cuff is placed around the limb just above the elbow. Depending on how thick the fur is, it may not be necessary to clip the leg – as long as good contact is made then an accurate reading should be obtainable. The Doppler probe is held over the ventral carpal area (ensuring that coupling gel is used to increase contact), and the cuff inflated. Inflation of the cuff will effectively stop any blood flowing through the blood vessels.

**Table 8.5**  Blood plasma liver related parameters in the healthy rabbit

| Parameter | Value in a healthy domestic rabbit |
|---|---|
| Aspartate transferase | 10–99 IU/L |
| Creatinine kinase | 140–372 IU/L |
| Gamma glutamyl transferase | 0–18 IU/L |
| Lactate dehydrogenase | 132–252 IU/L |
| Triglycerides | 0.3–1.7 mmol/L |
| Cholesterol | 0.2–2.0 mmol/L |
| Glucose | 5.5–8.2 mmol/L |
| $\beta$-Hydroxybutyrate | <1 $\mu$mol/L |
| Bile acids | 10–50 $\mu$mol/L |

As the cuff is gradually deflated, blood pumped out by the heart during systole will be able to pass through the blood vessels and this movement of blood will be detected by the Doppler. The pressure reading at this point should be noted (this is the systolic reading). Deflation of the cuff continues and there will come a point when blood moving through the cardiovascular system during diastole will be able to pass through the blood vessels and will again be heard via the Doppler. The pressure reading at this point should then be recorded. To ensure accuracy in these results, this procedure should be repeated two or three times (depending on the cooperation of the patient) and the average taken. Alternatively the cuff may be applied above the hock on a Lindley and the Doppler probe applied to the vertral surface of the metatarsal area.

A pulse oximeter may be applied to the central ear artery or the ventral base of the tail during anaesthesia. $pO_2$ stay above 97% assuming that there is good contact between the probe and the blood vessel. More information about pulse oximetry can be found in Chapter 6.

### 8.5.3  ECG

An electrocardiogram (ECG) can be used to examine a number of cardiac abnormalities including cardiac hypertrophy, conduction abnormalities and abnormal rhythms.

An ECG may be carried out on a rabbit which is sedated/anaesthetised for another purpose such as radiography, or can be carried out on a conscious rabbit. If attempting to obtain an ECG for a conscious rabbit,

**Table 8.6**  Reference blood pressure values

| Mean arterial pressure | 80–91 mm Hg |
|---|---|
| Systolic pressure | 92.7–135 mm Hg |
| Diastolic pressure | 64–75 mm Hg |

From Reusch (2005).

**Table 8.7** Electrode placement for an ECG

| Colour | Location |
| --- | --- |
| Red | Right forelimb |
| Black | Right hindlimb |
| Yellow | Left forelimb |
| Green | Left hindlimb |

the rabbit should be held on someone's knee or on a table, in sternal recumbency. Electrodes should be attached to the rabbit in a similar fashion to that for dogs (see Table 8.7), just behind the elbows and at a point halfway between the stifles and the hocks. Due to high heart rate a paper speed of 50 mm/second should be used, rather than 25 mm/second, and a deflection of 2 cm/mV. See Table 10.3 for normal ECG values (lead II) for healthy rabbits.

### 8.5.4 Syringe feeding

Due to the glutinous nature of many critical care supportive food, a large bore syringe (usually a non-Luer fitting, 50 mL syringe) should be used. Five to ten millilitres may be syringed into the side of the mouth at a time, allowing the rabbit to swallow in between administrations. A maximum of 15–20 mL at one sitting should be given. If in doubt, err on the side of caution and give more frequent small amounts.

### 8.5.5 Nasogastric/orogastric tube placement

Orogastric tubes may be used to deflate the stomach in cases of gastric dilatation or may be used to administer food/medication orally on a single occasion. Nasogastric tubes are more likely to be used to administer food long-term and they will be left in place.

Placement of the nasogastric tube can be carried out in a conscious or anaesthetised patient. Where conscious then local anaesthetic should be applied topically to the nasal mucosa. Small tubes (4–8 French) specifically designed for use in rabbits should be used wherever possible. Pre-measurement of the tube from the nares to the level of the seventh rib should be carried out prior to insertion. Local anaesthetic is applied to the tube and sprayed deep into the nose, using a latex catheter attached to the syringe ($\sim$0.2 mL). The end of the tube may be sutured or glued to the top of the head, midline. An Elizabethan collar may need to be applied to prevent the rabbit removing the tube.

### 8.5.6 Use of Elizabethan collars

There is much controversy over the use of Elizabethan collars in rabbits. This can be useful to prevent animals removing nasogastric tubes or stitches following surgery. However, they will also prevent the patient from carrying out caecotrophy. This is probably a situation where common sense should prevail. If a rabbit is anorexic and is not carrying out caecotrophy, then using a collar to retain a nasogastric tube in place is not causing any new problems. However, using a collar in a healthy animal to prevent suture removal following elective surgery would not be advisable.

### 8.5.7 Nasolacrimal cannulation

Cannulation of the nasolacrimal duct may be required to flush material such as pus through or to place contrast material in the duct during a radiographic work-up. Rabbits have a large, single ventral punctum, into which a 23-gauge latex catheter can be placed. The catheter should be attached to a 2-mL syringe containing saline or a saline antibiotic combination and then flushed through as shown in Figure 8.2.

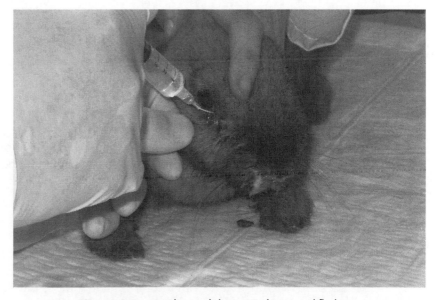

**Figure 8.2**  Nasolacrimal duct cannulation and flushing.

---

> **Box 8.4   Equipment required for urethral catheterisation**
>
> 1. KY gel (Johnson & Johnson)
> 2. 2.5–4 French Teflon-coated catheter
> 3. 10 mL syringe
> 4. Three-way tap
> 5. Collecting bowl

## 8.5.8 Cystocentesis

It is preferable to carry out cystocentesis in a rabbit which is sedated, although it is possible to carry this out in a conscious rabbit. The rabbit should be held on its back and an area clipped and surgically prepared from the pubis to the umbilicus and laterally to a region level with the hindlimbs. The rabbit will be held so that the bladder can be approached from a cranial to caudal direction so that as the bladder contracts it slips off the needle rather than tearing. A 23- to 25-gauge, 5/8″ needle is used on a 5–10 mL syringe. A three-way tap is useful to allow urine to be drained off without removing the needle from the rabbit.

## 8.5.9 Urethral catheterisation

Urethral catheterisation of the male rabbit requires a very small catheter. Female rabbits are slightly easier to catheterise than males, as they have a larger urethral opening, just inside the entrance to the reproductive tract. The perineal area should be cleaned with dilute chlorhexidine and dried prior to catheterisation. As for cystocentesis, most animals will be sedated for this procedure. Male rabbits should be held in dorsal recumbency and females in ventral recumbency with the hind legs drawn out behind them. Equipment required is listed in Box 8.4.

## 8.5.10 Taking skin samples

Skin samples can be collected for examination from rabbits, in exactly the same way as that for cats and dogs. Some more information about this is given in Table 8.8.

**Table 8.8** Collection of skin samples

| Sample | Comment |
| --- | --- |
| Coat brushing | Examine for evidence of fleas (flea dirt), lice, cheyletiella |
| Tape strip | Examine plain under microscope for evidence of cheyletiella and lice |
| Hair plucking | Examine proportion of anagen and telogen hairs |

# References

Orem, D.E. (1991) *Nursing: Concepts of practice* 4th edn, Mosby. St Louis.

Reusch, B. (2005) Investigation and management of cardiovascular disease in rabbits. *In Practice* 27:418–425.

Roper, N., Logan, W.W. and Tierney, A.J. (1996) *The Elements of Nursing: A Model for Nursing Based on a Model of Living*, 4th edn, Churchill Livingstone, New York.

# Specific Aspects of Medical and Surgical Nursing

## 9.1 Introduction

### 9.1.1 Drug toxicity

Drugs of the penicillin family, particularly the potentiated penicillins such as amoxicillin clavulanate, but also ampicillin- and amoxicillin-containing preparations, should not be used due to their ability to cause an enterotoxaemia with *Clostridia* spp. gut overgrowth. This may result in a fatal diarrhoea.

The same is true of many of the cephalosporin family and the macrolide family such as clindamycin, lincomycin and erythromycin.

## 9.2 Dental disease

### 9.2.1 Presentation and causes of dental disease

Dental disease is extremely common in captive rabbits. Dental problems may present with salivation and anorexia, through to jawbone swellings from root elongations of cheek teeth, to full-blown abscesses. Overgrown teeth may be obvious as with incisor malocclusions or may be hidden from external view as with cheek teeth malocclusions. Dental problems may affect other parts of the head, such as creating abscesses behind the globe of the eye, or affecting the lumen of the tear duct as it runs over the cheek teeth and around the maxillary incisor roots, causing pus to appear at the eye or nares.

Causes of dental disease can be hereditary defects such as a shortened rostrocaudal length of skull, trauma to teeth or jaws, and dietary deficiencies. The two most commonly cited dietary deficiencies include a lack of suitable abrasive foodstuffs for dental wear and a lack of calcium and vitamin D3 for proper jawbone mineralisation.

Rabbits have adapted over thousands of years to survive on a diet consisting of predominantly grass. Grass, of the meadow variety, is very high in silicates. These are abrasive compounds of silica, the chief mineral in sand, and are naturally very wearing. Rabbit's dental growth has thus evolved to cope with this. Even if the rabbit is not wearing its teeth down, they continue to grow at several millimetres per week. In addition, with a reduced abrasive diet, less vigorous chewing needs to be performed. As the rabbit's mandible is narrower than its maxilla, the only way the whole surface of the opposing sets of cheek teeth will wear evenly is by the lateral movement of the mandible across the maxilla. In less abrasive easier chewed diets, this happens less effectively, and so the outer/buccal edges of the mandibular cheek teeth wear, and the inner/lingual edges of the maxillary cheek teeth wear, causing sharp points to form on the tongue side of the mandibular teeth (see Fig. 9.1) and the cheek side of the maxillary. These points grow, the teeth tilt, and the mandibular teeth then cut into the tongue and the maxillary teeth into the cheeks, leading to deep ulcers, pain and anorexia. These

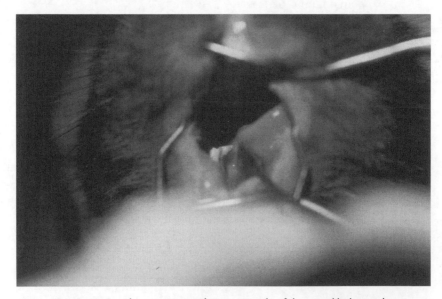

**Figure 9.1** Sharp points on the tongue side of the mandibular teeth.

problems are exacerbated in diets poor in calcium and vitamin D3 where poor jaw mineralisation allows increased movement of the roots of teeth as pressures are applied to their crowns, so 'tipping' the teeth further and more easily.

Root elongation is another feature of dental disease. The mandibular cheek teeth roots can push through the ventral aspect of the mandible, which may be felt as a series of lumps underneath the angle of the lower jaw. In the maxilla, the roots of the last two cheek teeth can push into the orbit of the eye, causing ocular pain and watering of the eye. All of the maxillary cheek teeth roots can cause blockage or strictures of the tear duct that runs in the bone above them. Roots that push through the jawbones can lead to abscessation, which may then involve further bone deposition by the body as the rabbit attempts to wall off the abscess.

Incisors may overgrow due to elongation of the cheek teeth as the growth of the latter teeth pushes the mouth open wider. The maxillary incisors are tightly curved, whereas the mandibular incisors are more gently curving. If the mouth is slightly forced open, the maxillary incisors no longer close rostral to the mandibular ones, and overgrowth ensues. The maxillary incisors curl back and into the mouth like rams horns, the mandibular incisors grow up in front of the nose. Root elongation may also occur with incisors with maxillary root elongation causing constriction of the tear duct that bends around them. This leads to inflammation and infection of the tear duct, which back dams and appears as a milky white discharge at the eye, known as dacrocystitis. This is often misdiagnosed as a primary conjunctivitis.

Overgrown incisors should never be clipped using nail clippers as this can cause fractures and splintering of the enamel, exposing the pulp and allowing infection to enter the tooth, as well as being painful. Instead they should be barred with a dental drill.

### 9.2.2 Nursing of dental disease

Prevention is the key. With some breeds, dental problems may be inevitable, and this should be explained to owners preferably before they purchase. All of the shorter nosed breeds, such as dwarf Netherland, and lops are susceptible owing to the shortened diastema and potential altered cheek tooth bite plane.

Dietary advice is essential – a good quality, largely grass-based diet is preferable. This can take the form of fresh grazed grass, good quality hay or dried grass products as well as proprietary grass pellets that are balanced for growth, particularly with reference to calcium and vitamin

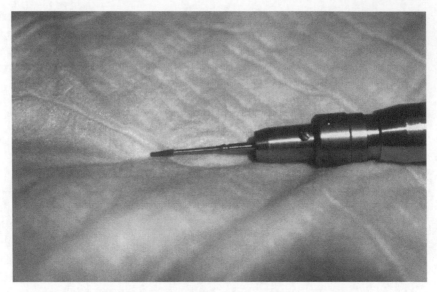

**Figure 9.2** A straight drill handpiece used to burr overgrown teeth.

D3 levels. Access to unfiltered natural sunlight, particularly during the juvenile growth phase, is also to be highly recommended for vitamin D3 synthesis.

If dental disease is already present then the options are limited. Regular burring of the affected teeth is often necessary. This should preferably be performed using straight drill handpieces of a dedicated dental unit (see Fig. 9.2). Radiographs of the head to look for root elongation are also important to provide information on the extent of the disease and whether abscesses are starting to form. Antibiotics and extractions of teeth may also be needed. Incisor extraction is now a relatively routine procedure if severe malocclusion has occurred (see Figs 9.3 and 9.4). Rabbits can manage well without incisors, provided food is offered in bite-sized portions, the rabbit can manipulate food items into its mouth perfectly well with its lips.

Where a rabbit is presented in poor condition, where anorexia has been present for a number of days or more, assisted feeding may be required. It is then vital to rehydrate the rabbit and provide much needed calories before attempting to anaesthetise or sedate the patient for dental work. In addition, many rabbits with dental disease will have a degree of gut stasis where the normal complicated peristaltic and antiperistaltic waves of the gut are reduced or have stopped altogether. A nursing plan will be required prior to anaesthesia and dental treatment to ensure success. This should ensure that the following points are addressed (see Box 9.1).

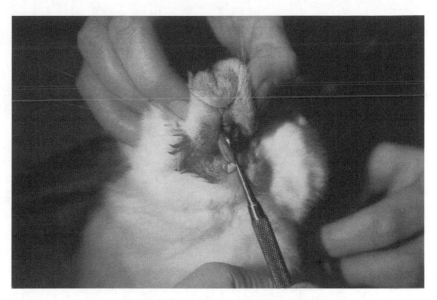

**Figure 9.3**   Extraction of incisor teeth.

If abscesses are present, it may be necessary to flush wounds with antiseptic on a daily basis. Most abscesses are best treated in rabbits by surgical excision as the pus produced is extremely thick and does not drain easily. Where this is not possible, then the abscess may be opened

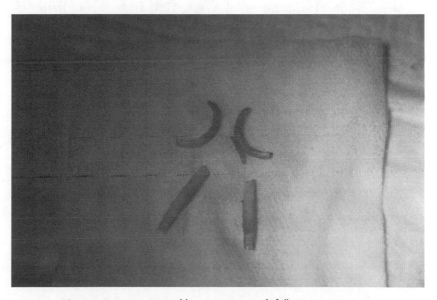

**Figure 9.4**   Upper and lower incisor teeth following extraction.

---

**Box 9.1  Outline of a nursing protocol for dental disease**

- Fluid therapy is administered (see Chapter 6)
- Analgesia is administered (see Chapter 6)
- Syringe feeding or a naso-oesophageal tube (see Chapters 4 and 10) is placed to allow food to be administered to attempt to correct energy and nutritional deficits
- Correct calorific requirements are calculated and divided over the course of a day
- Gastrointestinal (GI) prokinetics are administered to restart peristalsis (e.g. metoclopramide, ranitidine and cisapride)
- Probiotics or transfaunation of healthy rabbit faeces to recolonise the GI tract with beneficial bacteria
- Antibiotic therapy where abscessation/infection is apparent (e.g. fluoroquinolones or trimethoprim sulphonamides in the first instance, although culture and sensitivity testing is always advisable)

---

and treated as an open wound or packed with antibiotic-impregnated polymethylmethacrylate beads.

## 9.3 Digestive diseases

### 9.3.1 Causes and presentation of gastrointestinal disease

*Hairballs*

As with cats, some rabbits will overgroom and this may lead to an abnormal build-up of fur in the stomach. It should be noted that some fur in the stomach is normal in the healthy rabbit. However, excessive fur build-up can result in a trichobezoar being formed, and this may be associated with progressive gastric hypomotility which can occur due to dysautonomia or periods of stress. The trichobezoar or dilated stomach may be palpated in the cranial abdomen. Causes of overgrooming include lack of fibre in the diet; parasitic skin conditions; dental disease; and intestinal discomfort/disease.

*Diarrhoea*

*Dietary* causes of diarrhoea can include a sudden change in diet, as with the feeding of an excess of leafy greens to a rabbit previously fed dry formulas. This will lead to diarrhoea. Other dietary factors include the type of food fed, with spoiled foods and foods such as part-fermented grass cuttings inevitably leading to diarrhoea.

*Iatrogenic* causes include the administration of certain antibiotics such as many penicillins and the macrolide family. These can kill off the 'good' bacteria of the gut, leaving bacteria such as *Clostridia spiriformae*. This bacterium is found in small quantities in the normal flora of the rabbit gut, but once it achieves a critical threshold level, it can release an iota toxin that is absorbed across the gut wall into the bloodstream. This results in toxaemia, with hepatic and renal necrosis ensuing. Other clostridia such as *Clostridium difficile* and *Clostridium perfringens* have also been implicated, although to a lesser extent (Perkins *et al.*, 1995).

*Bacteria* such as the *Escherichia coli* family are particularly common in young recently weaned rabbits. These can be a cause of sudden death in these cases due to release of another form of toxin known as an enterotoxin. Death may occur before any signs of diarrhoea. Other bacteria less commonly seen include *Clostridium piliforme*, the cause of Tyzzer's disease which affects rabbits in the 6- to 12-week-old age range. This can cause acute diarrhoea and sudden death or a more chronic wasting malabsorption problem.

*Parasitic* causes of diarrhoea include the coccidial parasites *Eimeria* spp. These are single-celled protozoal parasites that inhabit the small intestine and destroy its lining, causing diarrhoea and death in heavy infestations, but may simply cause poor growth and stunting in mild cases. It is usually a disease of young rabbits. The coccidia *Eimeria stiediae* is of particular importance in rabbits as it will also infest and damage the liver. Coccidial oocysts may be detected in the faeces by direct smears or sugar solution flotation methods as for cats and dogs.

Other parasitic causes of diarrhoea and digestive upsets include the stomach worm *Graphidium strigosum* and the small intestinal worm *Trichostrongylus retortaeformis*. These are usually only found in rabbits with access to the outside whereby they may pick up the eggs of these worms directly from wild rabbits' faeces or indirectly via passive spread from wild birds, etc. A large intestinal pinworm *Passalurus ambiguus* is commonly seen, but rarely causes disease. All of these worms' eggs may be detected in the faeces by flotation methods.

*Viruses* such as rotaviruses can cause diarrhoea in weaned rabbits around the age mark of 6 weeks. Young rabbits become infected when the immunity instilled from colostrums from their mothers wears off. Generally the diarrhoea is mild and self-resolving (Thouless *et al.*, 1996).

### Mucoid enteropathy

This is a condition commonly affecting 4- to 14-week-old rabbits that are intensively reared and its causal agent is not known. They become colicky and pass thick mucus instead of faeces. As a result they are often dull, lethargic and in abdominal pain. On examination at post-mortem the caecal and large intestinal contents are often dried out and impacted with a large plug of mucus being present in the colon. The causes of this condition are not well identified, but the feeding of a highly fermentable low-fibre diet does predispose many rabbits to this. In addition, some evidence now suggests that a primary gut dysautonomia may be responsible for some cases.

### Intestinal dysautonomia

This is where a malfunction of the autonomic nervous system supplying the intestines results in a disruption of the normal peristaltic and antiperistaltic waves of contraction. Associated with this is often a profound bradycardia (<100 bpm), mydriasis, reduced tear production, urine retention and collapse of the affected rabbit. It was first reported in the UK by Whitwell and Needham (1996) in Belgian hares (which are confusingly rabbits and not hares) and mimicked 'mucoid enteropathy'. The intestinal dysfunction results in caecal impaction and often aspiration pneumonia. This is a condition that can only be diagnosed accurately by post-mortem as not all cases result in degenerative changes (chromatolysis) of autonomic nerve ganglia such as the mesenteric or celiac ganglia.

### Obstructive intestinal disease

Occasionally rabbits may develop an intestinal blockage associated with either a trichobezoar or some other foreign body. Diets including locust beans or dried peas can also be dangerous for this reason.

The rabbit may present with gastric dilatation due to a build-up of saliva/fluid and gas. It will not generally induce vomiting as the cardiac sphincter of the stomach in the rabbit is usually very tight and will not allow this. In addition, the deterioration of the patient is usually very rapid where a small intestine or stomach outflow obstruction occurs. Gastric dilatation may also occur as a result of the mucoid enteropathy condition, although in this case it tends to occur more gradually.

## 9.3.2 Nursing of gastrointestinal disease

*General nursing of gastrointestinal disease*

General nursing of the rabbit with gastrointestinal (GI) disease may be formulated as a nursing protocol (see Box 9.2).

In the case of specific disorders the following treatments may also be given:

*Specific nursing of trichobezoars*

Administration of supportive fluid therapy, gastric lubricants such as liquid paraffin, and keratinolytic preparations such as the enzyme

---

**Box 9.2   Outline of a nursing protocol for gastrointestinal disease**

- Start fluid therapy (see Chapter 6) even if diarrhoea is not ob-served as fluid may be trapped in the bowel by ileus. This should be by the intravenous or intra-osseous routes where intestinal disease is suspected.
- Ensure the rabbit is kept somewhere warm and with dimmed lighting away from stressors as many young rabbits with diar-rhoea are often in a very fragile state.
- Consider potassium supplementation if severe chronic diarrhoea is present (see Chapter 6).
- Administer analgesia where bloat or other painful conditions appear present (see Chapter 6).
- Protect the perineal and ventral body surface from scalding and infection from any diarrhoea – apply petroleum-based ointments (e.g. Vaseline®).
- Collect any diarrhoea or faeces passed for possible analysis.
- Assist feeding (see Chapters 4 and 10), ensuring sufficient calories are fed and particularly where diarrhoea has been associated with diet or iatrogenic causes, sufficient fibre is fed – *but only when obstructive bowel disease has been ruled out.*
- Use of prokinetics such as metoclopramide, ranitidine and cis-apride – *but only when obstructive bowel disease has been ruled out.*
- Use of probiotics or transfaunation of caecotrophs from a healthy rabbit to recolonise the gut flora.

papain (commonly found in pineapple juice) have all been advocated. Oral fluids and liquid paraffin certainly can help lubricate through smaller trichobezoars. Analgesia is advised for any intestinal/gastric discomfort, but the true cause of the overgrooming should be determined to prevent re-occurrence. Surgical removal of hairballs is fraught with difficulties as these individuals are often poor anaesthetic and surgical risks.

### Specific nursing of dietary diarrhoea

Medication may not be necessary. However, where acute severe diarrhoea is seen the use of anti-diarrhoeal compounds such as loperamide hydrochloride (Lomotil®) at 0.1 mg/kg orally, two to three times daily (although this is obviously not licensed for use in rabbits), has been advocated.

### Specific nursing of toxaemias

If toxaemia is suspected, often no amount of medication can save the rabbit, although shock doses of short-acting corticosteroids such as methyl prednisolone at 30 mg/kg intravenously may be tried.

For the *E. coli* family, the use of fluoroquinolones such as enrofloxacin at 5–10 mg/kg daily is advised. Oral cholestyramine (Questran®) may be used to 'mop up' further enterotoxins and prevent their absorption from the gut at 0.5 g/kg as a 2 g in 20 mL water solution.

### Specific nursing of gastrointestinal parasites

For coccidial problems the use of a trimethoprim sulphonamide drug at 48 mg/kg daily for 7 days is advised. The dosage should be repeated 7 days after the end of the initial course for a further 7 days to ensure removal of any dormant stages in the gut. This therapy has some effect against the hepatic coccidia *E. stiediae* although other drugs such as toltrazuril have more effect (see subsection 9.3.4). Good hygiene with regular cleaning of substrate and bedding material to reduce environmental contamination is essential to prevent re-infection.

Many intestinal worms such as *P. ambiguus* may not require treatment at all. Where large numbers are seen or where a trichostrongyle worm is present then these may be treated with ivermectin at 0.2 mg/kg or with fenbendazole at 20 mg/kg, once daily repeating the dosage on 4–5 consecutive days.

*Specific nursing of mucoid enteropathy and dysautonomia*

It may be possible to nurse a rabbit through mucoid enteropathy, and suggestions have been made that it is possible in cases of dysautonomia (Harcourt-Brown, 2002). Supportive therapy involving intestinal prokinetics, analgesia and liquid paraffin to aid softening of any colonic impactions can help. These should be combined with aggressive intravenous or intra-osseous fluid therapy and provision of a warmed, quiet and dimly lit environment to further support the patient. In both cases, however, the prognosis is poor.

*Specific nursing of intestinal obstructive disease*

Initial management should ensure rapid intravenous or intra-osseous fluid access for management of shock and analgesia and a rapid diagnostic work-up to confirm the diagnosis. Treatment is clearly a surgical procedure and carries a high risk in rabbits as peritonitis is common.

## 9.3.3 Causes and presentation of liver diseases

*Hepatic coccidiosis*

As mentioned in 'Diarrhoea' under subsection 9.3.1, the coccidial parasite *E. stiediae* can infect the liver of young rabbits and so induce hepatitis, resulting in ascites, poor weight gain and jaundice. Gamma glutamyltransferase elevations are associated with hepatobiliary disease rather than hepatocellular damage and therefore have been associated with conditions such as hepatic coccidiosis by *E. stiediae*.

*Hepatic lipidosis (fatty liver syndrome)*

Hepatic lipidosis is seen most commonly in overweight indoor rabbits that go through a period of anorexia or food withdrawal – similar to the situation seen in cats. However, as they are herbivores, rabbits withstand the absence of insulin far more easily than cats do and so a period of anorexia can be much more deleterious to rabbits. In rabbits the major energy source is absorbed in the form of volatile fatty acids from the caecum and during digestion of the caecotrophs. The liver maintains the blood levels of volatile fatty acids at a constant level despite the dietary fluctuations and is also responsible for converting them into lipids.

If starvation occurs the body's homeostatic mechanisms kick in, gluconeogenesis occurs from body fat mobilisation, producing free fatty acids that are taken to the liver. Ketones are then generated from free fatty acid metabolism and these enter the tricarboxylic acid (TCA) cycle. Acetoacetate is the parent ketone body, and the liver is unable to convert it back to acetoacetyl-coenzyme A which can enter the TCA cycle for gluconeogenesis. Most of acetoacetate is converted to $\beta$-hydroxybutyrate allowing transport around the blood, but a significant proportion stays as acetoacetate and acetone – both of which also have severe depressive effects on the central nervous system. All of the ketones create acidosis when present in excess. Rabbits appear unable to cope with even mild levels of ketoacidosis.

However, it is known that stress can also increase fat mobilisation in overweight rabbits. Studies showed that minor invasive procedures such as saline injections induced an increase in plasma free fatty acid and glycerol levels in obese rabbits (Lafontan and Agid, 1979). In addition, a high fat diet increases the risks of ketonaemia and so ketoacidosis in individuals who undergo anorexia as opposed to rabbits fed on a low-fat diet (Jean-Blain and Durix, 1985). Finally, it is well known that pregnant does between the days of 24 and 30 are highly insulin resistant (McLaughlin and Fish, 1994), adding to the likelihood that they will develop pregnancy ketosis.

So why does the liver become overburdened with lipids? The rate-determining step for the transport of lipids away from the liver is the liver's ability to synthesise the protein moiety of the lipoprotein required to remove lipids from hepatocytes that have been transported there due to a period of anorexia. The longer the anorexia, the worse the lipid mobilisation and the more the liver is swamped with lipids and free fatty acids. The lipids affect hepatocyte function and make them less able to successfully perform the TCA cycle, which is further exacerbated by an absence of glucose in the bloodstream. Once the liver has become lipidotic, the kidneys frequently follow suit.

The early stages of hepatic lipidosis may be imperceptible. As most cases are triggered by a period of anorexia, the main clinical signs to look out for are a reduction in food intake and faecal output. This should be taken seriously in all cases, and any rabbit anorexic for 12 hours or more (6–8 hours in pregnant does) should be given assisted feeding.

As the condition progresses, the rabbits become less and less responsive to its surroundings and external stimuli. Eventually they become comatose, hypoglycaemic, acidotic and die of liver and kidney failure. There is no liver-specific leakage enzyme in the rabbit; therefore, diagnosing hepatic damage in early stages is difficult. The liver leakage enzymes aspartate aminotransferase (AST), lactate dehydrogenase (LDH) and creatine kinase (CK) are measured together. AST is found in the liver and skeletal muscle; LDH in liver, cardiac and skeletal muscle; and CK only in skeletal muscle. Therefore, in cases of liver damage, AST and LDH may both be elevated but CK should remain within normal bounds. In most cases with hepatic lipidosis, there are elevations in the triglycerides and cholesterol levels as well as liver leakage enzymes. There may also be hypoglycaemia in severe cases, and levels of $\beta$-hydroxybutyrate will be elevated where ketosis is present.

Serum proteins may also be elevated, with general elevations in alpha-2 and beta globulins, particularly beta-1 globulins with beta-2 lipoprotein increases.

### Viral haemorrhagic disease

See 'Viral haemorrhagic disease' under subsection 9.4.1 for further information on this systemic disease, which can cause extensive liver necrosis.

## 9.3.4 Nursing of liver disease

For nursing of hepatic coccidiosis the use of trimethoprim sulphonamide drug is less effective. However, toltrazuril has been shown to be effective at reducing the severity of the disease when given in the drinking water at 25 ppm for 2 days and repeated again after 5 days (Peeters and Geeroms, 1986). For general liver supportive nursing the points listed in Box 9.3 should be considered. In addition, owners should be forewarned that even 12 hours of anorexia is a serious situation, particularly in pregnant does and overweight, elderly rabbits.

Anabolic steroids may be used (0.5–1.0 mg/kg once) to stimulate appetite and stop catabolism. Supplements such as choline, inositol, 'milk thistle' and L-carnitine may all be used to support liver function and promote lipid removal from hepatocytes. Lactulose has been used to alter the bacterial flora of the gut and reduce toxin production that the liver has to detoxify.

# 9.4 Respiratory diseases

## 9.4.1 Causes and presentation of respiratory disease

### Pasteurellosis and associated bacteria

The bacterium most commonly involved is *Pasteurella multocida* and causes 'rabbit snuffles' (see Fig. 9.5). It is commonly found in the airways

---

**Box 9.3  Outline of a nursing protocol for liver disease**

- Aggressive nutritional support is essential as early in the course of the disease as possible (see Chapters 4 and 10)
- Aggressive fluid therapy avoiding lactate-containing fluids, which require hepatic metabolism (see Chapter 6)
- The correction of any disease which may have initiated anorexia should then follow – these may be many and varied from dental disease, to renal disease, to gastric hairballs
- Treat hepatic coccidiosis with TMP/sulphonamides or toltrazuril
- Prokinetic medications such as cisapride, metoclopramide and ranitidine should be used but only where obstructive GI disease has been ruled out
- Use of nutraceuticals such as milk thistle, L-carnitine, inositol or drugs such as lactulose may help liver function

---

of apparently healthy rabbits, but it can lead to severe upper airway disease, with a purulent oculonasal discharge, and the characteristic wet, matted fur of the fore paws. This can lead to a pneumonia and septicaemia with the death of the rabbit, or may result in chronic abscessation of the lungs. It may also be associated with middle ear disease resulting in torticollis/vestibular disease. Poor housing, with damp,

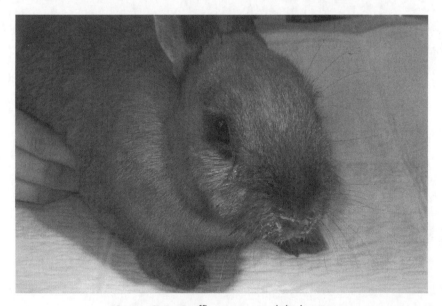

**Figure 9.5**  Snuffles – note nasal discharge.

ammonia-laden bedding can irritate the airways and allow rapid infection to occur. Dental disease and myxomatosis are other factors. Similarly, overcrowded hutches and concurrent disease elsewhere in the body may lower immunity.

In addition, other bacteria such as *Bordetella bronchiseptica* and *Staphylococcus* spp. may be associated with upper respiratory tract disease in the rabbit.

### Viral haemorrhagic disease

This is a calicivirus and has been in the UK since at least 1992. It does not exclusively cause respiratory disease but often causes a rabbit to die suddenly with a foamy haemorrhagic discharge from the nares. It is a systemic disease however and as such it will attack all organs within the body, particularly the lungs, digestive system and liver. It causes haemorrhages throughout the body by inducing disseminated intravascular coagulation. It is spread via contact and is stable in carcases for as long as 3 months in the wild and up to 1 month outside the host (Henning *et al.*, 2005), and is generally 100% fatal in non-vaccinated animals, often producing death with no obvious clinical disease. Post-mortem reveals widespread internal haemorrhage. Young rabbits over 2 months of age are most at risk. Interestingly, rabbits less than 4 weeks of age if infected do not show clinical signs of disease and develop a lifelong immunity. Those between 4 weeks and 2 months of age become increasingly at risk of developing the disease.

### Foreign bodies

Blades of grass or pieces of hay or straw may become lodged in one nasal passage. They may be seen projecting from the nostril or may not be visible but the rabbit may be showing signs of irritation and head shaking, a unilateral nasal discharge or repeated sneezing. There is also likely to be a degree of dyspnoea as rabbits are nasal breathers.

## 9.4.2 Nursing of respiratory diseases

For infectious disease, particularly where bacterial respiratory disease is suspected, then culturing, identifying and sensitivity testing the organism involved, and then administration of appropriate antibiotics is necessary where possible (see also Box 9.4). Fluid therapy is useful as excess respiratory secretions can lead to dehydration. Cleaning of the nares is important as rabbits are nose breathers. Consequently, the use

> **Box 9.4 Outline of a nursing protocol for respiratory disease**
>
> - Oxygen therapy if breathing is laboured or cyanosis is seen
> - Fluid therapy (see Chapter 6)
> - Cleaning of the nares is important as rabbits are nose breathers
> - May require nasolacrimal duct flushing if heavy oculonasal discharge
> - Mucolytics (drugs which break up the mucus) such as bromhexine hydrochloride (Bisolvon) at 1 mg/kg as either the injection or the oral powder is helpful. Steam inhalant baths are also useful to help break up the pus in the nasal passages
> - Nebulisation of antibiotics or mucolytics such as *N*-acetylcysteine to help break up respiratory secretions may also be useful
> - Antibiotics against *Pasteurella* spp. in particular useful (e.g. fluoroquinolones and TMP/sulphonamides)
> - Use of anti-inflammatories such as meloxicam or carprofen
> - Assisted feeding may be needed (see Chapters 4 and 10)

of mucolytics (drugs which break up the mucus) such as bromhexine hydrochloride (Bisolvon®) at 1 mg/kg as either the injection or the oral powder is helpful. Steam inhalant baths are also useful to help break up the pus in the nasal passages.

There is no treatment for viral haemorrhagic disease. Infection is almost invariably fatal to domestic rabbits. Prevention is possible with the oil-adjuvanted 'killed' vaccine Cylap® (Websters) dosed once annually subcutaneously.

Foreign bodies such as blades of grass or hay can be removed manually, although a rigid endoscope may be required where the foreign body is deeply implanted.

## 9.5 Skin diseases

### 9.5.1 Causes and presentation of skin disease

*Ectoparasites of rabbits*

**Mites**

*Cheyletiella parasitivorax* infestation produces a dense, white scurf, chiefly along the dorsum, starting usually around the nape of the neck and spreading outwards and caudally. Tufts of fur may be easily removed with the dandruff attached to their base. The condition may not appear pruritic, although in severe cases rabbits will self-traumatise. *C. parasitivorax* is a large mite, with an obvious waist when examined microscopically. The mouthparts have claws, and the ends of the legs possess combs rather than suckers. It is a potential zoonosis with bites appearing in the classical clusters of three (breakfast, lunch and dinner).

*Psoroptes cuniculi* is the ear mite of rabbits. It irritates the lining of the canal making it weep serum which dries in brown crusts within the ear canals and in severe cases may obliterate the lumen completely. The mites may be seen with the naked eye giving a pepper and salt appearance. Secondary bacterial ear infections which can lead to vestibular disease are serious sequels to infestation. The mite has a classical *Psoroptes* spp. form with pointed mouthparts and conical suckers to the ends of the legs when examined microscopically.

*Leporarcus (Listrophorus) gibbus* is a non-pathogenic fur mite of rabbits and therefore causes little or no disease. It is an oval mite with short legs, and so may be distinguished from *Psoroptes* spp. and *Cheyletiella* spp. on the clinical signs and the absence of a 'waist', conical suckers and combs on the end of its legs.

*Neotrombicula autumnalis* is the harvest mite. This is not a true parasite but the juvenile (six-legged as opposed to the adult eight-legged) bright orange red mite. It can be seen in rabbits with access to the outdoors or to hay/straw. It causes irritation of the skin surface chiefly over the palmar/plantar aspect of the feet, the face and ears. Its typical orange-red colour is visible to the naked eye and its six-legged form distinguishes it from other mites.

All of the above mites are surface dwelling, rather than burrowing mites. They may therefore be harvested for identification using a flea comb, or a Sellotape® strip applied to the affected area and then stuck to a microscope slide for examination.

Burrowing mites are uncommonly found in rabbits, the two main ones being *Sarcoptes scabei* and *Noetedres* spp. They appear similar to the forms found in other mammals such as cats and dogs, with intensely pruritic skin lesions, and are diagnosed after skin scrapings and examination microscopically.

**Lice**

*Haemodipsus ventricosis* is uncommon in domestic rabbits and belongs to the sucking (Anoplura) family. It is slender and often blood filled, and may cause significant anaemia in kits.

### Fleas

The rabbit flea is *Spillopsyllus cuniculi* and is the chief vector for transmitting myxomatosis. It tends to concentrate around the ears of the rabbit and may be distinguished from the cat and dog flea by the presence of obliquely arranged genal ctenidium. These are the fronds which line the mouthparts of the flea, and which are horizontal in the cat and dog flea.

### Blowfly strike

This horrible condition is common in outdoor rabbits in the summer months. It is particularly a problem in rabbits which have perineal soiling due to urine scalding or diarrhoea. The flies involved include the blue, black and green bottle families. These are the primary instigators of the disease, laying their eggs on the skin of the rabbit. In warm conditions these eggs hatch into larvae within 2 hours, and these immediately start to burrow into the rabbit away from the light.

### Other parasites

Another parasite known as *Coenurus serialis*, which is the intermediate host for the adult tapeworm of dogs (*Taenia serialis*), may form large fluid-filled cysts containing the scolices of the tapeworm in subcutaneous sites on the rabbit (see Colour Plate 24).

### *Viral skin infections*

### Myxomatosis

In naïve rabbits this condition is invariably fatal. However, in those rabbits with some immunity or where vaccination has been performed without the intradermal injection of the vaccine as well as the subcutaneous deposition, this may produce crusting nodules on the skin of the nose, lips, feet and base of the ears (see Colour Plate 25). In some rabbits, death will still occur up to 40 days after initial signs but many will recover. The acute form of myxomatosis as mentioned above is usually fatal and will produce oedema of the periocular region, the base of the ears and the anus and genital openings. It attacks the internal organs as well over a course of 5–15 days.

The myxomatosis virus is a member of the poxvirus family, and is transmitted by biting insects, chiefly fleas (principally the rabbit flea *S. cuniculi*), but mosquitos and lice may also provide a source of infection.

### Herpesvirus

There are two forms of herpesvirus affecting rabbits. One causes few if any physical signs, while the other may produce red lesions over the face and dorsum as well as damaging internal organs and leading to the death of the rabbit. There is no vaccine or treatment for these viruses.

## *Bacterial skin infections*

Rabbits form firm abscesses due to the thick consistency of rabbit pus. These are common in the head region where they are invariably associated with dental disease. The bacteria involved are often *P. multocida* and *Staphylococcus aureus* although after prolonged antibiotic treatment, many anaerobic bacteria will flourish.

'Blue fur disease' is caused by the bacteria *Pseudomonas aeruginosa*, which can produce a blue green pigment giving the condition its name. It is common in outdoor rabbits or those kept in damp conditions favouring *Pseudomonas* bacterial growth. It will infect damaged skin, such as occurs in the dewlap area of many lop breeds, where wet skin chafes.

Rabbit syphilis due to the bacteria *Treponema cuniculi* affects the anogenital area, the nose and lips, producing brown crusting lesions (see Figs 9.6 and 9.7). These may progress over the face. The bacterium is thought to be passed from doe to young during parturition, and may be sexually transmitted from buck to doe and vice versa. It is not infectious for humans.

## *Fungal skin infections*

The two commonly seen forms are the cat and dog ringworm *Microsporum canis* which will fluoresce under Wood's lamp light, and the environmental *Trichophyton mentagraphytes* which does not. The lesions are dry, scaly, often forming grey plaques appearing over the head initially, but then spreading to the feet and rest of the body. Brushings of the lesions and culturing them onto the usual dermatophyte medium is advised for definitive diagnosis.

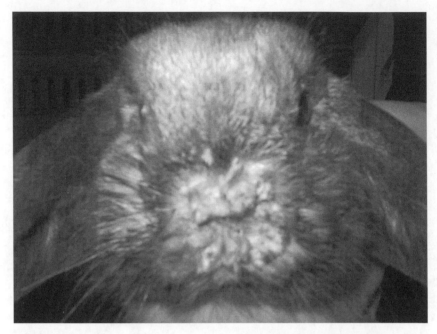

**Figure 9.6** Crusting around the nose in a case of syphylis. Courtesy of Ross Allan (Pets 'n' Vets).

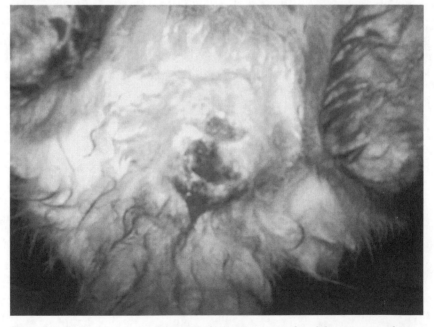

**Figure 9.7** Crusting around the genital area in a case of syphilis. Courtesy of Ross Allan (Pets 'n' Vets).

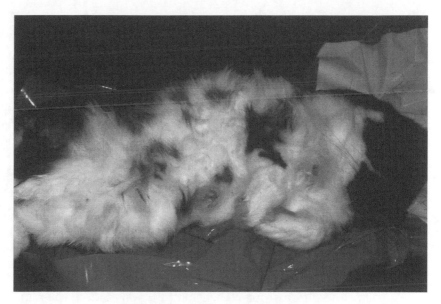

**Figure 9.8** T-cell cutaneous lymphoma.

## Skin cancers affecting rabbits

Subcutaneous lipomas are common in overweight older rabbits. Others include squamous cell carcinomas, particularly in white furred breeds kept outdoors, on their nose and ear tips where the fur is thinnest, lymphosarcomas in local lymph nodes, T-cell cutaneous lymphoma (see Fig. 9.8) and cancers or the hair follicles known as trichoepitheliomas. The lipomas and trichoepitheliomas are relatively benign and may be surgically removed. The others are more malignant and carry a guarded prognosis. Metastasis of other neoplasms to the skin, such as uterine adenocarcinomas, have also been seen by this author.

## Managemental problems

Rabbits are as prone to neglect as any other species. Particular problems occur in the fine and long-haired breeds such as the Angoras. This breed has especially fine fur, which mats easily, particularly when bedded on straw, hay or shavings. Owners of these breeds will need to be advised to keep them on paper or wire mesh and to groom their rabbit once or even twice daily. Even then, when the Angora moults in the spring and autumn, the chances are the coat will become matted. This can lead to dermatitis underneath the matted areas.

Overgrown claws are another common feature in rabbits, particularly hutch, kept rabbits with little access to the outside. Claws should be regularly assessed and, if necessary, trimmed on a 4- to 6-week basis. Overgrown claws can lead to lateral twisting of digit joints and deformity of the foot.

Perineal soiling is frequently seen. It may be due to faecal soiling from diarrhoea or inability or lack of desire to consume the caecotrophs which are softer than the faecal pellet. In addition, urine scalding is common, especially in older rabbits with spinal arthritis/spondylosis, which prevents them from positioning correctly to urinate. It is also a problem in lop breeds that have excessive folds of skin around the urogenital area.

Bacterial pododermatitis or 'sore hocks' is another often environmental or management problem. This is where sores appear just distal to the hocks due to pressure necrosis and infection. These may become so severe as to result in damage to the flexor tendons or even osteomyelitis. There are many causes including obesity, lack of space to exercise, soiled bedding, breed predisposition (rex breeds are more prone as they lack guard hairs), arthritis and abrasive floors.

### 9.5.2 Nursing of skin diseases

For general nursing plans for managing skin disease please see Table 9.1. Vaccination for myxomatosis is possible and is a live-attenuated vaccine which makes use of the Shope papilloma virus. This similar virus stimulates immunity against myxomatosis, but because it is not myxomatosis there is no danger of it causing the disease in rabbits. Vaccination occurs every 6 months in high-risk areas, such as outdoor-kept rabbits in the country or once yearly for indoor-kept town rabbits. The vaccine is administered as nine-tenths of the dose subcutaneously, and one-tenth given intradermally. The latter is important to provide the best possible systemic and cutaneous immunity so helping to prevent the cutaneous form of myxomatosis.

## 9.6 Cardiovascular diseases

### 9.6.1 Causes and presentation of cardiovascular diseases

*Arterial wall calcification and arteriosclerosis*

This occurs in rabbits fed excess amounts of vitamin D3 and calcium in their diets, although there may well be other aetiologies including

**Table 9.1** Outline of a nursing protocol for skin disease

| Skin complaint | Nursing protocol |
|---|---|
| Mites and lice | • Ivermectin at 0.2 mg/kg by subcutaneous injection on 2–3 occasions at 7–10 day intervals. Topical spot-on preparations now available in the UK for rabbits.<br>• For *C. parasitivorax* it may be necessary to increase the dose to 0.4 mg/kg due to the superficial nature of this mite.<br>• *Psoroptes* spp. can cause very infected and sore ears and analgesia with antibiotics may be required (see Appendix 1 for dosages). |
| Fleas | • Topical permethrin and imadocloprid spot-on are available commercially to kill adult fleas in the UK. |
| Blowfly strike | • For blowfly strike, prevention is better than cure, and treatment of any urine scald or diarrhoea is the first action which should be taken.<br>• The use of pupal development-inhibiting drugs such as cyromazine prevents the L1 'maggot' from developing into the L2 which is the stage which causes tissue damage.<br>• The provision of a fine fly proof mesh over any openings to the hutch should also be considered as is the use of permethrin spot-on preparations.<br>• Once parasitised, the rabbit will need analgesics such as meloxicam (Metacam®) at 0.3 mg/kg, covering antibiotics such as enrofloxacin (Baytril® 2.5% injectable), fluid therapy and often sedation with Hypnorm® to remove the maggots. Spraying the area affected with ivermectin diluted 1:10 with propylene glycol (being sure to keep the overall dose below 0.4 mg/kg) or injecting the rabbit with 0.4 mg/kg ivermectin once subcutaneously will help kill the maggots. |
| Viral | • Vaccines are available for the prevention of myxomatosis.<br>• Treatment of myxomatosis is supportive and involves fluid therapy, NSAIDs, assisted feeding and intensive nursing.<br>• Cutaneous form of myxomatosis does not generally need any treatment although anti-inflammatories may be given to reduce swelling and pain. |
| Bacterial | • Soft tissue abscesses – surgical excision of the enclosed abscess is best as antibiotics do not penetrate well into the thick capsule of the abscess or the glutinous pus inside.<br>• Non-excisable abscesses are, therefore, difficult to treat although packing the abscess with antibiotic-impregnated polymethylmethacrylate beads has proved useful.<br>• Treatment of blue fur disease may be performed with enrofloxacin dose of 5–10 mg/kg daily for 5–7 days and/or topical silver sulfadiazine cream.<br>• Treatment of rabbit syphilis may be performed with 24 mg/kg (40 000 IU/kg) of penicillin once weekly on 2–3 occasions.<br>• Great care should be taken with penicillin in rabbits as it may lead to a fatal diarrhoea, but at the above dosages no adverse effects have been seen.<br>• It is advisable to place the rabbit onto a probiotic (Entrodex® or Avipro®) and encourage hay/roughage consumption. |

*(continued)*

**Table 9.1**   (*Continued*)

| Skin complaint | Nursing protocol |
|---|---|
| Fungal | • Oral griseofulvin at 25 mg/kg twice daily for up to 4 weeks is effective for dermatophytes (ringworm).<br>• Care should be taken not to use this in pregnant does as this drug is teratogenic (the same should apply for staff handling the medication).<br>• Topical enilconazole (Imaverol®) at a 1:50 dilution applied every other day for up to 3–4 weeks. |
| Neoplastic | • Surgical excision where discrete tumours are present. |
| Managemental | • Provision of absorbant bedding underneath a deep layer of straw to keep the rabbit off the urine area is advised for mild cases of scald.<br>• Cage and rabbit hygiene are essential on a daily basis to prevent blowfly strike and secondary bacterial skin infections.<br>• In severe cases housing the rabbit on a suspended mesh floor so the urine and faeces drop through, as well as treating any underlying condition should be considered.<br>• Remove soiling of the perineum at least daily. This may require bathing but avoid excessive use of water as this can lead to maceration of tissues.<br>• Use barrier petroleum-based ointments.<br>• For bacterial pododermatitis surgical debridement of the area with systemic and topical antibiotics and analgesia is required.<br>• In addition, address cause of problem (e.g. obesity, arthritis and soiled bedding).<br>• Dressings may be applied to sores with aqueous gels to encourage healing but many are poorly tolerated by rabbits. |

chronic renal failure (CRF). The calcium becomes deposited in the tunica media of the walls of the major blood vessels, reducing their elasticity and leading to increased blood pressure. This may be seen radiographically with the aorta, subclavian arteries and sometimes renal vessels being commonly affected. This can lead to increased blood pressure, heart failure and clinical lethargy with weight loss and signs associated with heart failure in later stages.

### Cardiomyopathy and valvular disease

Heart disease is relatively common in domestic rabbits. Cardiomyopathy is more frequently seen in giant breeds of rabbits, although the cause is as yet unknown but may be associated with a genetic inherited component. Stress due to high stocking densities/too small environmental space is known in rabbits to lead to cardiomyopathies (Weber and Van der Walt, 1975). It is, however, possible for any systemic infectious disease to lead to inflammation of the heart muscle (myocarditis) and subsequent scarring of tissues, which can lead to a cardiomyopathy. Marini *et al.* (1999) have shown that respiratory tract *Pasteurella* spp. infections as well as a coronavirus infection and vitamin E deficiency can cause this. Pakes and Gerrity (1994) have also suggested that encephalitozoonosis can be a cause of cardiomyopathy. Finally, it is known that certain drugs, such as ketamine and xylazine combinations, have led to myocardial infarction and fibrosis which may lead to cardiomyopathy (Marini *et al.*, 1999).

Endocardiosis valvular defects are seen in older rabbits. These are accompanied by an audible murmur on auscultation and can result in congestive heart failure.

### Congestive heart failure

This is the end stage of cardiac disease and may be caused by any of the above aetiological agents. Radiographs show an enlarged heart with pulmonary oedema, although pleural effusions are sometimes seen with right-sided failure. Ascites and liver congestion may also be seen radiographically and ultrasonographically. On auscultation there may be audible murmurs and usually a tachycardia with increased respiratory noise. Clinically the rabbit is usually more lethargic, often anorexic, and may also suffer from GI stasis.

## 9.6.2 Nursing of cardiovascular diseases

Where congestive heart failure is present, the patient should be handled minimally and stress levels reduced as far as possible. Supplementary oxygen therapy is also advisable before attempting supportive medication. Diuretics such as furosemide (see Appendix 1) and thoracocentesis where required are advisable.

Thoracocentesis can be performed consciously as with the cat with the rabbit in sternal recumbency. The lateral chest wall is clipped of fur and briefly surgically scrubbed. A butterfly catheter of 23–25 gauge is attached to a 10 mL syringe via a three-way tap. The needle is inserted between the sixth and seventh ribs from caudal to cranial halfway between the sternum and thoracic spine, and fluid is drawn off. The same should be repeated with the other side of the chest.

Placement of a nasal oxygen catheter may provide more rapid and effective oxygen therapy (see Chapter 10). Long-term use of angiotensin-converting enzyme (ACE) inhibitors such as benazepril (Girling, 2003a)

> **Box 9.5 Outline of a nursing protocol for cardiovascular disease**
>
> ● Minimise stress, dim lighting reduce noise levels
> ● Provide supplementary oxygen – if necessary place a nasal oxygen catheter (see Chapter 10)
> ● Plan for the following:
>   ○ Radiography and ultrasonography (see Chapter 7)
>   ○ Possible thoracocentesis
>   ○ Intravenous catheter placement (see Chapter 8)
>   ○ Drug therapy (furosemide, ACE inhibitors; see Appendix 1)
>   ○ If severe bradycardia is present administer glycopyrrolate (see Chapter 10)

can be used to lower blood pressure and reduce the pressure on the heart. For further nursing protocols see Box 9.5.

## 9.7 Nervous system diseases

### 9.7.1 Causes and presentation of nervous system disease

For spinal and traumatic causes of neurological disease see section 9.9.

*Vestibular disease*

This can also be referred to as torticollis. One cause is encephalitozoonosis, others include tumours or infarcts of the hindbrain and more commonly *P. multocida* infection of the middle and inner ear. The bacteria gain access to the middle ear via the Eustachian canal or via a perforated eardrum in ear mite infestations. The balance centres in the inner ear and/or the hindbrain are affected, and the rabbit exhibits a head tilt of varying severity, which often worsens when stressed or handled (see Fig. 9.9), and a nystagmus. Many are unable to stand. Prognosis in these cases is poor and euthanasia should be considered. Pasteurellosis may be differentiated from encephalitozoonosis by blood sampling antibodies to *Encephalitozoon cuniculi* and by the fact that pasteurellosis tends to be associated with peripheral neurological disease and encephalitozoonosis with central. This means that the following clinical signs will be seen in encephalitozoonosis but rarely or not in pasteurellosis:

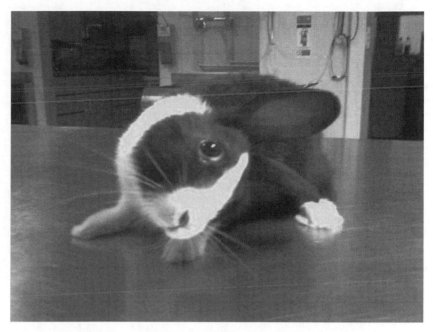

**Figure 9.9**  Head tilt in a rabbit with *Encephalitozoan cuniculi.*

- Intention tremors (indicative of cerebellar involvement)
- Depressed mental alertness
- Hemiparesis
- Presence of vertical and positional nystagmus (peripheral disease usually only horizontal or rotational nystagmus)

### Encephalitozoonosis

The microsporidian intracellular parasite *E. cuniculi* is common in many domestic rabbits. It is passed from rabbit to rabbit in the urine, gaining access via the oral or mucocutaneous route. It may be transferred from mother to young at the time of birth. It affects the kidneys and the central nervous system, and may remain latent for years, producing no clinical signs. Alternatively, paralysis of the hindlimbs, fitting, head tilts/vestibular symptoms anterior uveitis and blindness may be seen. Diagnosis is difficult to make in the live rabbit, as the only ante-mortem test so far available involves detecting the antibodies to the infection; therefore, a negative result is a definite negative, but a positive result in an otherwise healthy rabbit could merely suggest that the rabbit has been exposed to the parasite, but is not currently infected. Alternatively, the rabbit may be permanently infected. The development of laboratory tests which give an actual antibody titre has improved the diagnostic abilities of this test as this enables paired blood samples to be taken 2–4 weeks apart – a rising titre is strongly suggestive of recent infection.

### Floppy rabbit syndrome

This is a condition reported in pet rabbits that causes general muscle weakness and collapse. The aetiology is not currently known although possible causal agents have been suggested which include low blood potassium (hypokalaemia) – often associated with chronic renal disease; plant poisoning (see Appendix 2); other environmental toxins such as insecticides/herbicides (such as triazine weedkillers); lead poisoning and myasthenia gravis (Boydell, 2000). Some rabbits will recover with purely supportive therapy. Most are still able to eat and drink but have complete flaccid quadriparesis. 'Diagnosis' is made by ruling out other causes such as encephalitozoonosis or in the case of lead poisoning by measuring blood lead levels.

## 9.7.2 Nursing of nervous system diseases

The use of corticosteroids if hindbrain involvement has occurred is advised to reduce any swelling which may be impairing neurological function. However, it should be noted that corticosteroids can be immunosuppressive and rabbits are more sensitive to the side effects of corticosteroids than most, and this may allow the proliferation of organisms such as *E. cuniculi*.

In cases of suspected pasteurellosis, if culture is not possible, use a fluoroquinolone such as enrofloxacin at 10 mg/kg once/twice daily for 3–4 weeks. This sort of duration may be necessary before any improvement is seen. Surgery may be performed to open into the bulla affected by pasteurellosis to allow drainage. However, this author has found that due to the glutinous nature of the pus the success rate of this surgery is poor.

Treatment of *E. cuniculi* infection is difficult, but some recent work has suggested that the benzimidazole drugs, albendazole and fenbendazole, may be effective. Prognosis for recovery from neurological signs still has to be guarded.

General therapy of vestibular disease with drugs used in humans may be helpful. Examples include prochlorperazine (a phenothiazine) which is available in a liquid form and used for labyrinthitis in humans.

For further nursing protocols see Box 9.6.

---

**Box 9.6  Outline of a nursing protocol for neurological disease**

- Euthanasia in severe cases
- Minimise stress levels, noise to be reduced and lighting to be dimmed
- Minimise space provided for patients in cases of vestibular disease to prevent harm from falling/flailing around
- Assisted feeding (see Chapters 4 and 10)
- Fluid therapy (Chapter 6)
- Be prepared for intensive nursing to minimise scalding and soiling
- Plan for the following:
  ○ Radiography for bulla disease (see Chapter 7)
  ○ Intravenous catheter placement for medications for fitting (see Chapter 8)
  ○ Culture and sensitivity where possible (e.g. if ruptured tympanum is observed or bulla osteotomy performed)
  ○ Drug therapy: antibiotics for pasteurellosis; consider corticosteroids in severe cases controversial; fenbendazole for encephalitozoonosis; use of vestibular disease drugs from humans; use of benzimidazoles such as diazepam or midazolam where fitting occurs

---

## 9.8 Urinary and reproductive tract diseases

### 9.8.1 Causes and presentation of urinary tract disease

*Urolithiasis and cystitis*

This is a common problem in rabbits, due to their unusual method of controlling calcium levels in the body whereby they absorb all of the calcium they can from their diet, and then excrete any excess into the urine via the kidneys. The commonest urolith to form is the calcium carbonate crystal. This readily forms in the alkaline rabbit's urine, and is radio-dense, being seen to fill the bladder outline on radiography. Secondary bladder infections are common with severe calcium carbonate urolithiasis, as the crystals irritate the lining of the bladder, and secondary, often *E. coli*, infections result.

### Haematuria

The presence of red-coloured urine in the rabbit does not necessarily indicate haematuria as many red porphyrin pigments from the diet (particularly some leafy greens and beets such as beetroot) will be excreted in the urine. Causes of haematuria vary from cystitis, to uterine tumours and aneurysms, to kidney infections.

### Encephalitozoonosis

Infection of the kidneys with *E. cuniculi*, a protozoal single-celled microsporidian parasite, can cause severe scarring and damage. This parasite may also be responsible for various neurological signs (see section 9.7). The most common renal presentation is chronic renal disease due to a granulomatous interstitial and tubular degeneration.

### Acute renal disease

This is associated with a rabbit in good bodily condition, sometimes with a history of recent medication administration (e.g. nephrotoxic drugs such as the aminoglycosides or some non-steroidal anti-inflammatory drugs (NSAIDs)) or in does in late pregnancy with toxaemia or in obese animals which undergo a period of anorexia where fatty infiltration may occur (hepatic lipidosis may also be seen). Blood parameters will be elevated as for CRF, but there is often renal shutdown and anuria (see Chapter 8 for normal parameters). The main difference between acute and chronic failure is the loss of body condition and generally slower onset of debilitation and polydipsia/polyuria in chronic failure. Causes of acute renal failure (ARF) include drug toxicity (aminoglycosides, non-selective NSAIDs) and infections (e.g. pyelonephritis and glomerulonephritis and rarely *E. cuniculi* causing an interstitial nephritis) as well as fatty infiltration. The latter may be associated with ketosis with the presence of $\beta$-hydroxybutyrate as well as other ketones in the bloodstream. In addition, although unlikely, a bilateral ureteral obstruction or urethral obstruction may result in renal failure.

### Chronic renal disease

This is generally associated with similar signs observed in other mammals, e.g. weight loss, dehydration, loss of appetite, polydipsia and polyuria. In addition, a reduction in GI motility, with bouts of GI stasis and caecal impaction, may be observed. Urine produced is dilute with often a significant proteinuria (a mild proteinuria is normal in young rabbits; see Chapter 8 for normal urine results). An assessment of urine protein/creatinine levels can be made using in house kits designed for cats. Although no definitive normal values exist for rabbits, this author (Girling) and others use the cut-off range for cats as a reference point.

Soft tissue mineralisation may be seen in cases of CRF. Clinical anaemia may be present, and other clinical signs associated with specific conditions (e.g. neurological signs with *E. cuniculi* infection) may also be demonstrable.

Renal neoplastic lesions may present as CRF cases or may show other clinical signs depending on their spread. The most common neoplasm is renal lymphoma.

### 9.8.2 Causes and presentation of reproductive tract disease

#### Uterine adenocarcinoma

This is a common condition seen in does over the age of 4 years (see Fig. 9.10). Some authors have put the incidence at nearly 80%. The condition is fatal if not detected early as the tumour readily metastasises to the lungs primarily. Radiography of the chest is therefore advised if the condition is suspected to determine if spread has occurred. Spaying at 5–6 months of age is preventative providing all uterine tissue has been removed.

#### Venereal spirochaetosis

This is rabbit syphilis due to the bacteria *T. cuniculi*. The condition produces a tan-coloured crusting of the anogenital area and the nose and lips. It is transmitted sexually and from doe to kitten at the time of birth.

#### Pyometra

Uterine infections do occur in older does, and are often due to *E. coli* infections of hyperplastic endometrial tissues or uterine neoplasia. Renal damage can occur from *E. coli* infections and death from peritonitis should the uterus rupture is likely.

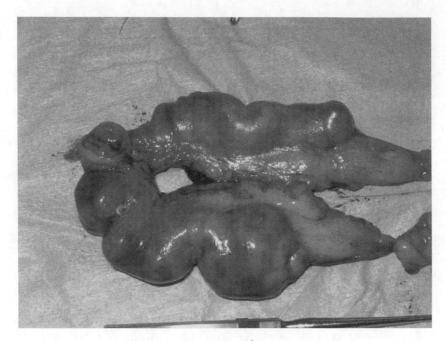

**Figure 9.10** Uterine adenocarcinoma.

## Mastitis

This is seen following pregnancy where the kittens are lost or in phantom pregnancy. The unused milk can become easily infected, particularly if the hutch/environmental conditions are poor. Many of the coliform type of bacteria involved will release endotoxins into the bloodstream causing rapid toxaemia, fever and death of the doe. Others may just cause severe mastitis with abscess formation.

### 9.8.3 Nursing of urinary and reproductive tract diseases

See Table 9.2 for a summary of treatment and outline of nursing protocols.

## Urolithiasis/cystitis

Reduction of calcium in the diet to reduce crystal formation is advised (see Chapter 4) with flushing of the bladder either surgically or via catheterisation to remove the worst of the crystal sludge. Samples taken for culture and sensitivity testing are advisable. Whilst awaiting results,

**Table 9.2**   Outline of a nursing protocol for urinary and reproductive tract diseases

| Urinogenital disease | Nursing protocol |
|---|---|
| Urolithiasis/cystitis | • Dietary restriction of calcium 0.6–1% dry matter (Lowe, 1998; Chapter 4)<br>• Analgesia (see Chapter 6)<br>• Management of urine scald likely around perineum (see Table 9.1 managemental) |
| Encephalitozoonosis | • Fenbendazole is the treatment of choice<br>• See subsection 9.7.2 for further treatment |
| Acute renal disease | • Fluid therapy (see Chapter 6)<br>• Verapamil use may be of help<br>• Treatment for encephalitozoonosis if diagnosed |
| Chronic renal disease | • Fluid therapy of an aggressive nature should be instituted (see Chapter 6)<br>• Dietary restriction of calcium (0.6–1% dry matter) to prevent soft tissue mineralisation (Lowe, 1998; Chapter 4)<br>• Anabolic steroids and vitamin B injections may be of some palliative help<br>• Use of benazepril may be helpful (Girling, 2003a)<br>• Treatment for encephalitozoonosis if diagnosed, although damage often already done and non-reversible |
| Uterine adenocarcinoma | • Preparation for radiography/ultrasonography to diagnose and determine if metastasis has occurred (see Chapter 7)<br>• Surgical spaying if caught early enough. This is one of the main reasons for recommending routine neutering of does at 5–6 months of age as this obviously prevents the condition<br>• Fluid therapy of an aggressive nature should be instituted (see Chapter 6)<br>• Analgesia and preparation for surgery (see Chapter 6) |
| Rabbit syphylis | • See Table 9.1 |
| Pyometra | • Stabilisation with fluids (see Chapter 6), and covering antibiotics such as enrofloxacin (see Appendix 1) are advised initially<br>• Surgical ovariohysterectomy should then be considered as soon as the doe is fit enough to undergo this procedure and the doe prepared for an anaesthetic (see Chapter 6)<br>• Fluid therapy of an aggressive nature should be instituted (see Chapter 6) |
| Mastitis | • Any abscesses present should be lanced and flushed out under sedation/anaesthesia if the doe is stable enough<br>• Swabs for bacteriological culture and sensitivity should be taken<br>• A broad-spectrum antibiotic such as enrofloxacin or trimethoprim sulfadiazine should be started (see Appendix 1)<br>• Antipyretics/analgesics such as meloxicam or carprofen (see Chapter 6 and Appendix 1)<br>• Fluid therapy of an aggressive nature should be instituted (see Chapter 6) |

a fluoroquinolone antibiotic is advisable. Analgesia and fluid therapy are also advised (see Chapter 6).

## Chronic renal failure

As with other mammals, reversal is not possible. Management is therefore based on limiting the levels of phosphorus (<0.5% dry matter) and calcium (<1%) in the diet – protein levels should already be relatively low on formulation diets. Fluid levels should be assessed and levels of water-soluble vitamins (B and C chiefly) should be maintained by supplementation. Treatment of potential GI ulceration with ranitidine (2 mg/kg PO every 12 hours) is advisable.

Work by this author (Girling, 2003a) and subsequent studies have looked at the use of ACE inhibitors, principally benazepril, to help maintain renal perfusion in these cases. Rabbits appear very sensitive to the hypotensive side effects of this drug, but doses of 0.1–0.2 mg/kg appear to be tolerated and prolong survival times with a lowering of urea, creatinine and phosphate levels seen, a stabilisation of blood albumin and a lowering of the hypertension seen with CRF. Weekly blood pressure monitoring is still advised in these cases (see Chapter 6).

Erlich *et al.* (1997) have also recommended using 8 mg/kg aspirin PO once daily in humans to prevent platelet agglutination and microthrombus formation in the renal arterioles, which significantly contributes to progressive renal fibrosis. Antacids such as ranitidine must be used in conjunction to prevent gastric ulceration.

Ongoing fluid therapy should also be considered with some authors recommending regular, daily subcutaneous injections of sterile crystalloid fluids at rates of 25–50 mL/kg split over the day.

Anabolic steroids may be used (0.5–1.0 mg/kg once) to stimulate appetite and stop catabolism and stimulate red blood cells' production in cases of chronic anaemia.

## Acute renal failure

If pre-renal failure is present then this should be corrected (i.e. when systolic pressure is less than 90 mm Hg) with crystalloids as a 15–20 mL/kg bolus slowly IV. If severe hypotension is present, combining this with 3–5 mL/kg of a colloid (e.g. Hetastarch®/Dextran®) at the same time is advisable.

After this, rehydration of the patient is necessary assuming maintenance values for rabbits are 80–100 mL/kg per day and deficits are calculated as for cats and dogs. The output of urine should be recorded every 3–4 hours. An easy method is to use pre-weighed absorbent pads under the rear of the rabbit and assume that every gram increase in weight is equivalent to 1 mL of urine. Insensible losses in the rabbit are assumed to be 1 mL/kg/hour. Ongoing fluid levels may therefore be calculated. Most rabbits with ARF will become 3–5% dehydrated each ongoing day of therapy and so extra fluids to counteract this should be given.

When fluids in are equivalent to fluids out (including insensible losses) and the blood urea nitrogen and creatinine levels have returned to their normal ranges, fluid therapy may be stopped assuming the patient is eating and drinking.

If hyperphosphataemia and hypercalcaemia are present then use phosphorus-binding agents (e.g. aluminium hydroxide 30–60 mg/kg PO every 12 hours).

Urinary tract infections should be treated with a fluoroquinolone, e.g. enrofloxacin 10 mg/kg once/twice daily in the first instance whilst awaiting culture and sensitivity results. If neurological signs are associated with ARF then treatment for *E. cuniculi* should be instituted whilst awaiting serological results (see section 9.7).

Treatment for fatty infiltration or the kidneys is discussed in 'Hepatic lipidosis' under subsection 9.3.3.

Removal of nephrotoxic medications and administration of antidotes such as vitamin B6 supplementation (5 mg/kg PO/SC) should be given where drugs such as gentamicin have been used.

Verapamil has also been used to treat acute renal ischaemia and may be of help in acute renal failure. It works as a calcium channel blocker and appears to protect the proximal tubules from ischaemic necrosis. Doses of 0.2 mg/kg SC every 8 hours have been used (Carpenter, 2005).

## 9.9 Musculoskeletal diseases

### 9.9.1 Causes and presentation of musculoskeletal disease

*Splayleg*

It is an inherited congenital disease whereby the kit cannot position one or more limbs underneath itself, instead the limb sticks out awkwardly. It is usually restricted to the hindlimbs. Severe cases cannot be treated and euthanasia should be considered. Some rabbits will cope with a degree of splayleg.

### Fractured/dislocated spine

This is a common condition in indoor reared, poorly fed rabbits. The close confinement leads to weakening of the bones and muscles due to disuse atrophy, and the absence of sunlight can exacerbate a vitamin D3 deficiency in a poor diet along with calcium deficiency creating metabolic bone disease. Osteoporosis occurs with spontaneous fractures often located in the lumbosacral area. Fractures of spinal vertebrae may be compression or complex type. In addition, younger individuals may show vertebral growth plate fractures.

Luxations and subluxations are also common in rabbits. This is particularly so when they have pre-existing osteoporotic conditions due to poor diets and lack of exercise, or when they are inappropriately handled without controlling their powerful hindquarters.

### Other fractures

The skeletal structure of the rabbit is delicate. Only 7–8% of the total body weight of the rabbit is composed of skeleton, compared with 12–13% in domestic cats. This is partly due to a decrease in the organic component of the bone matrix, which leads rabbit bones to be more brittle than their feline counterparts. This is seen in many rabbit fractures whereby complex fractures are common. Fractures of the tibia are often mid-shaft at the point where the cross section of the bone goes from triangular shaped proximally to oval distally. Femoral fractures are common and usually complex, occurring just proximal to the condyles at the point where the main quadriceps muscles attach.

### Osteoarthritis including spondylosis

In one study, three types of spinal lesions were observed in the rabbit (Green *et al.*, 1984). This produced a range of problems, which could result in spinal arthritis (spondylosis) along the whole length of the spine by 2 years of age, or may be seen mainly in the thoracic region in rabbits as young as 3 months (see Chapter 7). Developmental kyphosis and scoliosis of the spine also occurs and may place further pressure on the discs as well as making locomotion difficult. Spinal lesions in general may also reduce the ability of the rabbit to perform caecotrophy, and lead to scalding of the perineum due to an inability to position itself to urinate without soiling the ventrum.

Myelography may be performed using the L6/7 intervertebral space (Longley, 2005) can be used to look for partial or full disc rupture and spinal damage (see Chapter 7).

Osteoarthritis of all limbs is common in rabbits, particularly those over 4 years. It can be associated with sepsis in the case of pododermatitis certainly in younger rabbits.

### Nutrition muscular disease

This is a disease of young rabbits and is rarely seen in domestic rabbits. A suboptimal level of vitamin E in the diet (see Chapter 4) leads to generalised muscular weakness which may present as splayleg or as a rabbit that cannot right itself when rolled onto its back.

## 9.9.2 Nursing of musculoskeletal diseases

### Spinal injuries

Loss of pain sensation to the rear limbs is a poor sign as in cats and dogs, and euthanasia should be considered. Spinal surgery is possible in cases of fractures or where disc surgery is needed. However, little information is available in the literature to illustrate success rates of such treatment. NSAIDs can be of help where partial disc displacements or paresis is present (see Box 9.7).

### Fractures

Distal limb fractures can be initially stabilised with splints and padded dressings to prevent further soft tissue damage. Long-term use of dressings however does not work as rabbits tend to chew them out. Most limb fractures require surgical external fixation due to their complex nature, the often flattened cross section of the bones such as the femur and their brittleness. The exception is the tibia which is a more tubular-shaped bone and generally fractures in a more simple fashion.

### Osteoarthritis

Limiting excess body weight, encouraging gentle exercise and the use of NSAID analgesia is advised. Intra-articular injections of corticosteroids should be avoided.

---

**Box 9.7   Outline of a nursing protocol for musculoskeletal disease**

- There is no treatment for splayleg
- Limb fractures require surgical repair or application of light-weight fibreglass casts depending on their severity
- Dietary supplementation with calcium and vitamin D3 should be started, with gentle exercise to strengthen the bones. Care should be taken not to over-supplement (see Chapter 4)
- Use of NSAIDs in the short- and long-term for pain relief and management of spinal disease and osteoarthritis
- Physiotherapy of paretic limbs once any fracture/instability has been dealt with is of help to prevent further muscle wastage and pressure sores. Similar techniques to those employed in cats may be used
- Supplementation with vitamin E where nutritional muscular disease is suspected

---

*Nutritional muscular disease*

It is frequently not possible to treat this condition. However, if caught early enough, dietary supplementation of vitamin E and selenium may help (see Chapter 4 and Appendix 1).

## 9.10 Nursing of neonates

### 9.10.1 Fostering care

Rabbit kittens are difficult to artificially rear. Many females will not foster a strange doe's kittens, but does kept together, and lactating at the same time will often allow the suckling of the other's young. This is the best scenario if another known lactating doe is available. If not, as is often the case, hand rearing may be attempted. A rearing formula has been worked out (Okerman, 1994) as 25 mL of cows' whole milk to 75 mL of condensed milk and 6 g of lyophilised skimmed milk powder. A vitamin supplement may be added to this. The kitten is fed twice a day only, from 2 to 10 mL depending on the age. This should continue until the kitten is 2 weeks old when more and more good quality hay and pellets should be introduced, aiming to wean the kitten at 3 weeks.

> **Box 9.8   Conditions of geriatric rabbits**
>
> - Congestive heart failure
> - Dental disease
> - Neoplastic disease (e.g. uterine adenocarcinomas and fibrosar-
>   comas)
> - Osteoarthritis
> - Pododermatitis
> - Renal disease (chronic)
> - Urine scalding

The anogenital area should be stimulated with a piece of damp cotton wool after every feed to stimulate urination and defaecation for the first 2 weeks.

## 9.11 Nursing of the geriatric rabbit

Certain conditions are obviously more likely to be present in older rabbits. These include those listed in Box 9.8.

The nursing of the older rabbit should therefore take these conditions into consideration. This includes ensuring close monitoring of food intake, as assisted feeding is essential as mentioned before to prevent GI stasis and other conditions such as hepatic lipidosis.

In addition, many geriatric rabbits are already on medications such as NSAIDs for osteoarthritis amongst other things. This should be taken into consideration when deciding on further medication, e.g. further NSAIDs should be avoided if additional analgesia is required and antacids should be considered.

Extra padding and increased frequency of bedding change may also be required where there are concerns regarding soiling and skin infections such as pododermatitis.

## 9.12 Pre- and post-surgical nursing

### 9.12.1 Pre-surgical nursing

For pre-anaesthetic procedures see Chapter 6. All rabbit patients should of course be in a fit enough state, where possible, to undergo surgery.

If the rabbit is not, then postponement of the surgery until sufficient stabilisation can be achieved is advisable. This is particularly the case where anorexia is present and/or gut stasis. These can lead to hepatic lipidosis and other post-surgical complications if not addressed prior to surgery.

Surgical preparation of the patient for an operation should involve initially clipping the fur over the surgical site. This should be done in the preparation room as rabbit fur is very fine and otherwise gets everywhere. Care should be taken to avoid clipper rash as this is very common in rabbits and leads to increased likelihood of wound self-trauma after surgery. Scrubbing of the site for surgery should follow the same principles as for cats and dogs. However, care should be taken to avoid using excessive amounts of liquid and avoid using surgical spirit to reduce the cooling effects these create during the anaesthetic.

## 9.12.2 Post-surgical nursing

A rapid return to normal appetite is essential in rabbits to prevent postoperative complications such as intestinal ileus. This can be facilitated by ensuring good analgesia, adequate hydration and the use of reversible/quick recovery anaesthetics. In addition, providing the rabbit with a familiar foodstuff in its own bowl(s) is essential in many cases to reduce anxiety and rejection of food altogether. The patient may not be on the best diet for a rabbit when he/she comes into the surgery, but immediately after a surgical procedure and anaesthetic is not the time to start drastically altering it.

If dental surgery has been performed it may be necessary to hand-feed or syringe feed the rabbit with appropriate critical care and support formula diets (see Chapter 4). In addition, analgesia and prokinetic drugs that stimulate gut motility and so help prevent ileus and encourage appetite will often need to be used.

Management of any wounds should ensure they remain clean and free of discharge. Sutures are usually placed subcutaneously or intradermally (see Figs 9.11 and 9.12) to prevent the patient from chewing them out. However, the wound should be closely observed for signs of opening or for evidence of gnawing on behalf of the rabbit, which can occur uncommonly.

The use of dressings should be avoided as these are poorly tolerated by rabbits and can lead to gut impactions if eaten.

It is essential to monitor food and water intake and urine and faecal pellet output immediately after surgery. If there is any doubt about

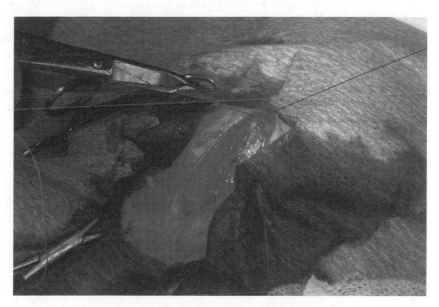

**Figure 9.11** Placement of subcuticular sutures.

appetite or thirst, then assisted feeding and fluid therapy (which is generally routinely advised after anaesthetics see Chapter 6) should be started. Similarly, if faecal output or urine output is not detected or is significantly reduced within the first 12–24 hours after surgery, assisted

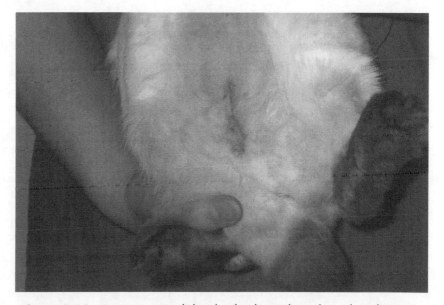

**Figure 9.12** Cystotomy wound closed with subcuticular and intradermal sutures.

---

**Box 9.9 Outline of a nursing protocol for post-surgical nursing**

- After recovery from anaesthesia, monitor heart rate and body temperature every 30–60 minutes for the first 3–4 hours
- Monitor wound for dehiscence and self-trauma
- Ensure adequate analgesia (use combination NSAID and opioid if severe pain; see Chapter 6)
- Monitor food and water intake closely in the first 12–24 hours – if in doubt:
  - ○ Assist feed (see Chapters 4 and 10) and
  - ○ Administer fluid therapy (see Chapter 6)
- Monitor faecal and urine output – if in doubt again:
  - ○ Assist feed (see Chapters 4 and 10)
  - ○ Administer fluid therapy and
  - ○ Administer intestinal prokinetics/antacids

---

feeding, intestinal prokinetics, analgesia and antacids and fluid therapy will again be essential (see Box 9.9).

# References

Boydell, P. (2000) Nervous system and disorders. In: *Manual of Rabbit Medicine and Surgery*, 1st edn (ed., Flecknall, P.), BSAVA, Quedgeley, Gloucestershire, pp. 57–62.

Carpenter, J.W. (2005) *Exotic Animal Formulary*, 3rd edn, Elsevier Saunders, Philadelphia.

Erlich, J.H., Holdsworth, S.R. and Tipping, P.G. (1997) Tissue factor initiates glomerular fibrin deposition and promotes major histocompatibility complex class II expression in crescentic glomerulonephritis. *American Journal of Pathology* 150:873–880.

Girling, S.J. (2003a) Preliminary study into the possible use of benazepril in the management of renal disease in rabbits. In: *Proceedings of the British Veterinary Zoological Society, Autumn Meeting*, Edinburgh, p. 44.

Green, P.W., Fox, R.R. and Sokoloff, L. (1984) Spontaneous degenerative spinal disease in the laboratory rabbit. *Journal of Orthopaedic Research* 2:161–168.

Harcourt-Brown, F. (2002) Digestive disorders. In: *Textbook of Rabbit Medicine*. Butterworth-Heineman, Edinburgh, pp. 249–291.

Henning, J., Meers, J., Davies, P.R. and Morris, R.S. (2005) Survival of rabbit viral haemorrhagic disease (RVHD) in the environment. *Epidemiology and Infection* 133:719–730.

Jean-Blain, C. and Durix, A. (1985) Effects of dietary lipid level on ketonemia and other plasma parameters related to glucose and fatty acid metabolism in the rabbit during fasting. *Reproductive Nutritional Development* 25:345–354.

Lafontan, M. and Agid, R. (1979) An extra-adrenal action of adrenocorticotrophin: physiological induction of lipolysis by secretion of adrenocorticotrophin in obese rabbits. *Journal of Endocrinology* 81:281–290.

Longley, L. (2005) Epidural catheterisation in rabbits. In: *Proceedings of the British Veterinary Zoological Society Spring Meeting*, Chester 2005, pp. 56–57.

Lowe, J.A. (1998) Pet rabbit feeding and nutrition. In: *The Nutrition of the Rabbit* (eds, Blas, C.D. and Wiseman, J.), CABI Publishing, Cambridge, pp. 304–331.

Marini, R.P., Li, X., Harpster, N.K. and Dangler, C. (1999) Cardiovascular pathology possibly associated with ketamine/xylazine anesthesia in Dutch belted rabbits. *Laboratory Animal Science* 49:153–160.

McLaughlin, R.M. and Fish, R.E. (1994) Clinical biochemistry and haematology. In: *The Biology of the Laboratory Rabbit*, 2nd edn (eds, Manning, P.J., Ringler, D.H. and Newcomer, C.E.), Academic Press, London, pp. 111–124.

Okerman, L. (1994) Breeding problems. In: *Diseases of Domestic Rabbits*, 2nd edn, Blackwell Publishing, Oxford, pp. 113–120.

Pakes, S.P. and Gerrity, L.W. (1994) Protozoal diseases. In: *The Biology of the Laboratory Rabbit*, 2nd edn (eds, Manning, P.J., Ringler, D.H. and Newcomer, C.E.), Academic Press, London, pp. 205–224.

Peeters, J.E. and Geeroms, R. (1986) Efficacy of toltrazuril against intestinal and hepatic coccidiosis. *Veterinary Parasitology* 22:21–35.

Perkins, S.E., Fox, J.G., Taylor, N.S., Green, D.L. and Lipman, N.S. (1995) Detection of *Clostridium difficile* toxins from the small intestine and caecum of rabbits with naturally acquired enterotoxaemia. *Laboratory Animal Science* 45:379–384.

Thouless, M.E., DiGiacomo, R.F. and Deeb, B.J. (1996) The effect of combined rotavirus and *Escherichia coli* infections in rabbits. *Laboratory Animal Science* 46:381–385.

Weber, H.W. and Van Der Walt, J.J. (1975) Cardiomyopathy in crowded rabbits. *Recent Advances in the Study of Cardiac Structural Metabolism* 6:471–477.

Whitwell, K. and Needham, J. (1996) Mucoid enteropathy in UK rabbits: dysautonomia confirmed. *Veterinary Record* 139:323–324.

## Further reading

Girling, S.J. (2003b) *Veterinary Nursing of Exotic Pets*. Blackwell Publishing, Oxford.

Meredith, A. and Flecknall, P. (eds) (2006) *Manual of Rabbits*, 2nd edn, BSAVA, Quedgeley, Gloucestershire.

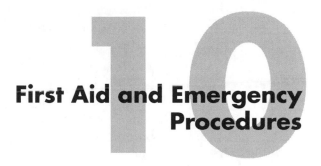

# First Aid and Emergency Procedures

## 10.1 Introduction

Emergency medicine is a challenging discipline and perhaps none more so than in some of the smaller patients that we deal with. Rabbits are often presented to veterinary practices and emergency clinics with acute ailments, many of which can lead rapidly to a life-threatening condition. Although specific information on emergency medication of the acutely collapsed rabbit is scarce, the medical approach should follow protocols already created for cats and dogs, but with some tailoring of the therapy based on the differing anatomy and biology of the rabbit. This chapter aims to provide the nurse with information on first aid, emergency therapy and stabilisation of the domestic rabbit.

## 10.2 First aid

The advice given to an owner will to a certain extent depend on the situation as presented by the owner over the telephone; however, there are some generic rules to advise in all circumstances and these include the following:

- Keep the rabbit still and warm (wrapping in a blanket/towel leaving the head free can be a means to achieve both of these aims)
- Keep the lighting dimmed and the noise levels down
- Remove the rabbit from any cage mates or open water bowls particularly if incapacitated

- Contact (if not already doing so) their local rabbit veterinary practice for further information

In certain specific situations other advice should be offered (see Table 10.1).

The same advice can be taken by staff within a veterinary practice should similar emergencies arise. For specific emergency protocols please see section 10.3.

**Table 10.1**  Telephone advice to owners in specific emergency cases

| Problem | Advice |
|---|---|
| Bite wounds | If the wound is on a limb, immobilise the limb. In all cases place a clean absorbent dressing over the wound and hold this in place. Do not advise owners to flush wounds as this may result in their inadvertently flushing debris and infection deeper into the tissues. Advise immediate veterinary assessment of the wound. If bleeding occurs then give appropriate advice as outlined below. |
| Bleeding wounds | Apply a clean cloth to the area and maintain moderate pressure In the case of badly bleeding wounds/arterial damage, advise the owner to apply a tourniquet above the wound if possible, tightening until blood flow stops. This should then be periodically released every 8–10 minutes for a matter of 30 seconds to 1 minute until arrival at the veterinary surgery. |
| Electric shocks | Isolate the power source involved first before removing the rabbit from the cabling/equipment. |
| Fitting/seizuring | Dim lighting and minimize noise levels and do not disturb until fitting ceases. However, if fitting continues beyond 4–5 minutes, it may be necessary to uplift the rabbit and travel to the veterinary surgery for further emergency treatment. |
| Fractures | The most likely recognised fractures will be limb fractures. The owner should be advised to minimise the lifting and movement of the rabbit until the limb can be immobilised. If the rabbit is still very active then restrict the rabbit to a small carrying cage or cardboard box and minimise noise and light levels to discourage activity until veterinary treatment can be provided. |
| Spinal injuries | If there is evidence of hind and or forelimb paresis or paralysis, spinal injuries should be considered as these are common in rabbits. Owners should be advised to keep the rabbit as still as possible by reducing lighting and noise levels. In addition, restricting the rabbit by placing solid bolsters, such as rolled towels, either side of its body to prevent rolling in transport is advisable. |
| Thermal burn | Immediate application of cold water for a period of 2–3 minutes is advised to minimise collateral tissue damage. Once cooled, the wound should then be covered with a dampened sterile/clean dressing until veterinary treatment can be performed. |

## 10.3 Emergency procedures

Traditional 'ABC' – airway, breathing and circulation – protocols already adopted for cats and dogs should be used in rabbits.

### 10.3.1 Emergency airway access and ventilation (A and B)

Immediate endotracheal intubation should be attempted if hypoxia is detected or cessation of breathing occurs.

If the rabbit is still breathing then endotracheal (ET) intubation may be achieved blindly. The rabbit is placed in sternal recumbency and its head is lifted vertically. The ET tube is then entered through the mouth and advanced in midline slowly. It is helpful to place your ear close to the end of the ET tube to listen for breathing sounds through the tube. The tube may then be quickly advanced into the trachea on inspiration. If a transparent ET tube is used then condensation from the rabbit's breath when the tube is over the glottis can be seen aiding intubation.

If the rabbit is no longer breathing then the blind technique becomes extremely difficult as no air sounds or condensation will occur. In these cases direct visualisation of the glottal opening is necessary. A laryngo-scope with a Wisconsin 0 paediatric blade or equivalent can be used to visualise the glottis (see Fig. 10.1) (Heard, 2004). The rabbit is placed in

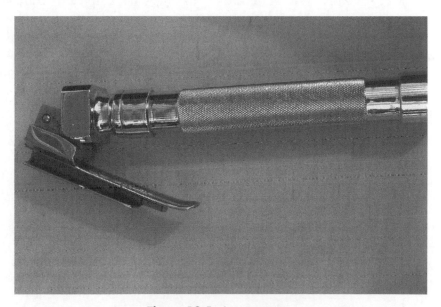

**Figure 10.1**  Laryngoscope.

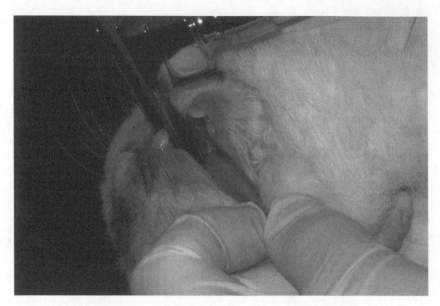

**Figure 10.2**   Insertion of laryngoscope into mouth of rabbit.

dorsal recumbency whilst carefully pulling its tongue out to one side of its mouth (see Fig. 10.2). The laryngoscope blade is inserted with the handle of the laryngoscope pointing vertically upwards so using the curved blade to further push the tongue upwards and away from the roof of the mouth. As the blade is advanced it is often necessary to gently push the soft palate away from the epiglottis as the latter normally sits above it, allowing nasal respiration. This then allows visualisation of the glottal opening. A guide wire is useful at this stage. These are plastic-coated flexible lengths of wire used in human medicine to aid intubation. It is inserted through the glottis first. Once in place, the ET tube is then slotted over the top of it and advanced along its length and so into the trachea. The guide wire is then withdrawn. An alternative technique may be used using a fine endoscope or needlescope. These are inserted into the lumen of the ET tube and so used as a sort of guide wire. The ET tube with scope is advanced into the glottis and then holding firmly to the ET tube the scope is withdrawn.

In some cases even direct intubation is not possible due to the narrow oral cavity and relatively large size of the tongue caudally or the presence of an obstruction such as a pharyngeal abscess or foreign body. It therefore may be necessary to pass a transtracheal catheter or perform a tracheostomy (see Colour Plates 26–33). Transtracheal catheters have been specifically manufactured for rabbits and are the same as over the

needle intravenous (IV) catheters. The principle is simple: the trachea
is grasped in one hand and the over the need catheter is inserted in between two tracheal rings into the lumen of the trachea. The inner needle
is then withdrawn and the catheter is secured in place. Tracheostomy is
relatively straightforward except in a few cases such as with some breeds
of rabbit, particularly in the doe, that have large dew flaps with plentiful
subcutaneous fat depots covering the trachea. Otherwise a longitudinal
incision is made over the trachea caudal to the larynx, followed by blunt
dissection onto the trachea itself in the same manner as for cats and
dogs. A 180° ventral incision in-between the tracheal rings, three–four
rings below the larynx, is made and an ET tube inserted. This may then
be attached to a breathing circuit for ventilation via a Luer adaptor. The
ET tube or catheter should be secured in place. This may be performed
either by suturing it to the surrounding skin or using a tie to tie around
the back of the neck.

Another alternative is the laryngeal mask. These are human paediatric
ET tubes with an inflatable cuff at their tip. The ET tube is blindly inserted
through the mouth until the tip is situated in the caudal oropharynx just
above the glottal opening. The cuff is then inflated and oxygen supplied
through the ET tube in the usual manner (see Chapter 6). Intermittent
positive pressure ventilation may be performed with this technique,
but it often results in inflation of the stomach with air that can in itself
impede respiration by pressure on the diaphragm. However, if voluntary
breathing is still present, this technique is very successful in this author's
opinion.

If direct or indirect intubation is not possible then the use of a tight-
fitting face mask connected to an anaesthetic circuit with a high flow
rate of oxygen (4–5 L) may be tried. Alternatively a face mask with an
Ambu bag attached may be used in a similar manner to force ventilate
the rabbit. Some authors have recommended moving the rabbit in a
see-saw manner alternatively head down and then up, so moving the
abdominal viscera backwards and forwards onto the diaphragm and
acting as a pump mechanism (Briscoe and Syring, 2004). This works
on the basis that most of the impetus for inspiration comes from the
flattening of the diaphragm rather than the outward movement of the
ribcage in the rabbit.

## 10.3.2 Cardiovascular support (C)

Direct cardiac massage by compressing the chest directly over the heart is
most effective in increasing thoracic pressure and forcing blood through

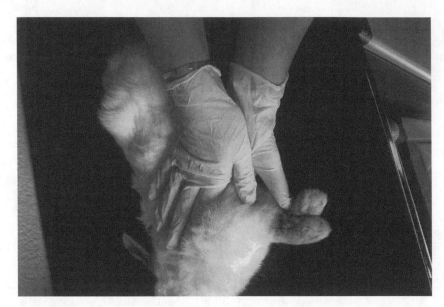

**Figure 10.3** Circumferential chest compression. (Originally published in *Vet Times*.)

the arterial vasculature in mammals less than 10 kg in weight (Henrik, 1992) with the majority of rabbits belonging to this category of mammal. Due to their rapid heart rates, compression rates of 100 bpm need to be achieved in rabbits; the technique recommended to maximise cardiovascular output is circumferential chest compression (see Fig. 10.3), as is used in human infants, where the chest is compressed over the heart from both sides at once (Costello, 2004).

Electrocardiogram (ECG) leads should be applied to the rabbit when a cardiac beat is felt or the heart restarted to identify any dysrhythmias. In cats and dogs the type of dysrhythmia detected during resuscitation has been associated with electromechanical dissociation, whereas in rabbits, profound bradycardia, ventricular asystole and ventricular fibrillation have been reported (Rush and Wingfield, 1992). Adrenaline may be used where no cardiac beat can be detected. It is preferably administered intratracheally if intubated or can be administered intravenously or via the intracardiac route if not. Intracardiac administration can be difficult due to the thin size of the ventricular walls and small size of the heart. In the case of fine ventricular fibrillation seen on an ECG trace, the use of adrenaline has been advocated to convert the electrical activity to coarse ventricular fibrillation, which is easier to convert to normal rhythms (DeFrancesco, 2000) (see Table 10.2 for dosages).

**Table 10.2** Emergency drugs used in rabbits

| Drug | Dosage and route |
| --- | --- |
| Adrenaline (1:1000 = 1 mg/mL) | 0.2–1 mg/kg IV, intratracheally |
| Carprofen | 1–4 mg/kg SC, PO q24 hours |
| Dexamethasone | 2 mg/kg IV (use with caution) |
| Diazepam | 1–3 mg/kg IV, IM |
| Doxapram | 2–5 mg/kg SC, IV, orally q15 minutes |
| Fluids | 100 mL/kg/day maintenance |
| Furosemide | 1–4 mg/kg IV, SC, IM |
| Glycopyrrolate | 0.02 mg/kg SC, IM |
| Lidocaine | 1–2 mg/kg IV; 2–4 mg/kg intratracheally |
| Midazolam | 0.5–2 mg/kg IV, IM, intranasally |
| Meloxicam | 0.3–0.6 mg/kg SC, PO q24 hours |

Adapted from Kottwitz and Kelleher (2003) and Flecknall (2006).
PO, per os; IM, intramuscularly; SC, subcutaneously; IV, intravenously.

Coarse ventricular fibrillation may be converted to normal rhythms by the use of cardiac massage as described above, or if the clinic has access to defibrillation devices then the use of these externally at 2–10 J/kg (starting at low energies and increasing if no response is achieved) (Costello, 2004). Greater success is achieved with defibrillation devices if three initial countershocks are applied at low energies.

Severe bradycardia is a common abnormality in the critical care rabbit. To convert this to normal rhythms, glycopyrrolate should be used (see Table 10.2) in preference to atropine as 60% of domestic rabbits possess serum atropinesterases, making atropine less effective (Okerman, 1994).

Lidocaine is rarely used in rabbits as ventricular tachycardia is uncommon. It definitely should not be used where atrioventricular blocks or severe bradycardia is seen which are the cardiac dysrhythmias more commonly seen in rabbits (DeFrancesco, 2000). Lidocaine may be administered intratracheally or intravenously if ventricular arrhythmias such as VPCs leading to ventricular tachycardia do occur.

Congestive heart failure as a result of cardiomyopathy and valvular insufficiency as well as atherosclerosis is also seen in rabbits and may present 'acutely' as an emergency. Treatment of congestive heart failure initially depends on the use of diuretics such as furosemide at 1–4 mg/kg IV, repeated every 4–6 hours as required. Angiotensin-converting enzyme inhibitors have been used in rabbits, but they are more susceptible to their hypotensive side effects than cats or dogs. Therefore, reduced dosages and regular monitoring of the systolic blood pressure using non-invasive techniques devised for cats are advisable (Girling, 2003).

In addition, as with cats and dogs, they should only be used after sufficient diuresis has been performed.

## 10.4 Emergency diagnostic procedures

### 10.4.1 Electrocardiogram

The ECG trace can provide valuable information upon which to base medication. In rabbits the standard three lead trace is the minimum requirement and is applied to the four limbs of the rabbit as one would to a cat or dog. It may however be necessary to file down the alligator clips as rabbit skin can be thinner than cats and dogs and so more prone to trauma. See Table 10.3 for some normal ECG trace values for rabbits.

### 10.4.2 Radiography and ultrasonography

Both techniques may be required where acute gastrointestinal signs are present, such as bloat, or visceral pain, or where evidence of limb fractures, paresis or paralysis is present, and should be performed when clinically safe to do so as part of a full clinical work-up. Further information on diagnostic imaging is provided in Chapter 7. Abdominal pain may be caused by renal calculi, obstructive and non-obstructive intestinal ileus and peritonitis. Spinal trauma such as luxations, fractures and dislocations may also be identified radiographically. Gradation of severity may be made as with cats and dogs. Acute treatment of spinal damage with anti-inflammatory drugs (see Table 10.2) and immobilisation with analgesia is advised particularly where concurrent paresis or

**Table 10.3** Normal ECG values (lead II) for healthy rabbits

| Parameter | Normal result | Notes |
|---|---|---|
| P-wave height | 0.1–0.15 mV | Deflection is low or negative in lead I and always positive in leads II and III |
| P-wave duration | 0.03–0.04 seconds | |
| P-R interval | 0.05–0.1 seconds | |
| QRS complex duration | 0.015–0.04 seconds | |
| R-wave amplitude | 0.03–0.39 mV | |
| Q-T interval | 0.08–0.16 seconds | Change of deflection of the T-wave from positive to negative or vice versa indicates myocardial hypoxia as with cats and dogs |

From Kozma *et al.* (1974) and Huston and Quesenberry (2004).

paralysis is present. Surgery may then be performed for collapsed discs or fractures in cats and dogs as required.

## 10.5 Intensive care

### 10.5.1 Fluid therapy

Fluid therapy is covered in more detail in Chapter 6. However, covered here is a brief outline of emergency fluid therapy for completeness. If the rabbit is dehydrated or hypovolaemic, shock doses of fluids should be administered. It should be noted that fluids should be avoided post-resuscitation in cases of cardiovascular arrest where there is no hypovolaemia/dehydration prior to the arrest as these fluids may decrease myocardial perfusion pressures and diminish overall nutrient delivery through the cerebral and coronary vasculature (Cole *et al.*, 2002).

The marginal ear vein, jugular vein, cephalic vein and lateral saphenous vein can all be used for IV catheter placement. Long-term (>2–3 days) use of the marginal ear vein may however cause sloughing of the ear tip, although in the author's experience this is relatively rare with careful venipuncture technique. Use of a topical local anaesthetic cream is recommended prior to placement.

Intra-osseous catheters may be placed into the proximal femur, in the trochanteric fossa, in a parallel direction to the long axis of the femur. Use an 18- to 23-gauge, 1–1.5 in. spinal or hypodermic needle. Analgesia should be employed (see Chapter 6) whenever placing an intra-osseous catheter as should prophylactic antibiosis.

Intra-osseous and intravenous fluid administration should be accurately titrated using syringe drivers rather than relying on drip sets, as even a small error in fluid administration may be proportionally more significant, considering the small size of many rabbits.

### 10.5.2 Analgesia

Many acute emergencies are associated with considerable pain, e.g. fractures, intestinal obstructions, pyelonephritis and renal calculi. In addition, if performing any invasive procedure, analgesia should be considered. The same care should be taken when using non-steroidal anti-inflammatory drugs in rabbits as is taken with their usage in cats and dogs, i.e. they should be avoided where renal disease or gastric/intestinal ulceration/perforation is suspected (see Chapter 6).

### 10.5.3 Critical care nutrition and prokinetics

The main aspects of rabbit nutrition are covered in Chapter 4. In this chapter, we cover the basics of critical care nutritional support as well as the problems of hypomotility of the gut.

Gastrointestinal stasis is a potential sequel for any rabbit presented with a life-threatening problem. Provided obstructive gastrointestinal diseases have been ruled out, the use of prokinetic medications such as cisapride, metoclopramide and ranitidine can be considered. Cisapride is becoming increasingly difficult to source at present but is an effective large bowel motility enhancer. Ranitidine acts to reduce acidity in the stomach which is beneficial as many rabbits with gastrointestinal stasis have multiple tiny ulcers of the stomach lining. Ranitidine has also some prokinetic effect and this is synergised by its combination with metoclopramide. Dosages of these three medications are given in Table 10.4.

Assisted feeding should be carried out in conjunction with the use of prokinetics. This can start off with solutions of easily absorbed essential sugars and amino acids (such as Critical Care Formula® Vetark Professional) either syringed into the mouth or delivered via a naso-oesophageal tube. As the rabbit improves clinically, this should be stepped up to use proprietary critical feeding formulas that provide some source of fibre such as Science Recovery® (Supreme Petfoods) or Critical Care for Herbivores® (Oxbow Pet Products) or vegetable-based baby foods (lactose-free varieties as many rabbits cannot digest lactose). The disadvantage of the baby foods is that they do not contain fibre and so have little or no prokinetic activity, although they do provide nutrients in an easily digestible form and so are preferred by this author earlier on in the course of nutritional support where providing sufficient calories to keep the patient going is essential.

The levels of energy required for a debilitated rabbit should approach that calculated for growing to lactating rabbits using the formula

**Table 10.4** Dosages of prokinetic drugs in rabbits

| Drug | Dose rate | Frequency of dosing and notes |
|------|-----------|-------------------------------|
| Cisapride | 0.5 mg/kg PO | 12 hourly (now difficult to obtain) |
| Metoclopramide | 0.5 mg/kg SC | 8–12 hourly |
| Ranitidine | 2–5 mg/kg PO | 12 hourly (in combination with metoclopramide acts to promote motility as well as reducing acidity) |

PO, per os; SC, subcutaneously.

$\text{MER} = k \times (\text{wt[kg]})^{0.75}$, where $k = 200$ for growth and 300 for lactation (Carpenter and Kolmstetter, 2000). Therefore for debilitation, the following daily energy requirement may be used:

$$\text{MER} = 250 \times (\text{wt [kg]})^{0.75}$$

It is essential to ensure the correct calorific levels are provided for the patient. This is due to fatty liver degeneration (hepatic lipidosis), another common, and often fatal, sequel to a negative energy balance situation in the rabbit.

Further help in promoting normal gut activity is to ensure the re-population of the intestinal flora. Transfaunation of caecotrophs from a healthy rabbit may aid the return of normal bowel function. This is where the caecotrophs (the dark green/brown sticky intermediate droppings) are taken from a healthy rabbit and then mixed into a slurry and gavaged or stomach tubed into the patient. The use of commercial probiotics designed for rabbits has also been advocated, and reduces the risk of transferring potential parasites and other agents to the debilitated patient.

# References

Briscoe, J.A. and Syring, R. (2004) Techniques for emergency airway and vascular access in special species. *Seminars in Avian and Exotic Pet Medicine* 13(3):118–131.

Carpenter, J.W. and Kolmstetter, C.M. (2000) Feeding small exotic animals. In: *Hill's Nutrition III* (eds, Lewis, L.D., Morris, M.L. and Hand, M.S.), Mark Mervis Institute, Marceline, Missouri, pp. 943–960.

Cole, S.G., Otto, C.M. and Hughes, D. (2002) Cardiopulmonary cerebral resuscitation in small animals: a clinical practice review. *Journal of Veterinary Emergency and Critical Care* 12:261–267.

Costello, M.F. (2004) Principals of cardiopulmonary cerebral resuscitation in special species. *Seminars in Avian and Exotic Pet Medicine* 13(3):132–141.

DeFrancesco, T.C. (2000) Cardiac emergencies. In: *Kirk and Bistner's Handbook of Veterinary Procedures and Emergency Treatment* (eds, Bistner, S.I., Ford, R.B. and Raffe, M.R.), WB Saunders, Philadelphia, pp. 54–61.

Flecknall, P.A. (2006) Anaesthesia and post-operative care. In: *Manual of Rabbit Medicine and Surgery*, 2nd edn (eds, Meredith, A. and Flecknall, P.), BSAVA, Quedgeley, Gloucestershire, pp. 154–165.

Girling, S.J. (2003) Preliminary study into the possible use of benazepril in the management of renal disease in rabbits. In: *Proceedings of the British Veterinary Zoological Society*, p. 44, November, Edinburgh.

Heard, D. (2004) Anesthesia, analgesia and sedation of small mammals. In: *Ferrets, Rabbits and Rodents: Clinical Medicine and Surgery*, 2nd edn (eds, Quesenberry, K.E. and Carpenter, J.W.), WB Saunders, St Louis, pp. 356–369.

Henrik, R.A. (1992) Basic life support and external cardiac compression in dogs and cats. *Journal of the American Veterinary Medical Association* 200:1925–1931.

Huston, S.M. and Quesenberry, K.E. (2004) Cardiovascular and lymphoproliferative diseases. In: *Ferrets, Rabbits and Rodents: Clinical Medicine and Surgery*, 2nd edn (eds, Quesenberry, K.E. and Carpenter, J.W.), WB Saunders, St Louis, pp. 211–220.

Kottwitz, J. and Kelleher, S. (2003) Emergency drugs: quick reference chart for exotic animals. *Exotic DVM*, 5.5 (November):23–25.

Kozma, C., Macklin, W., Cummins, L.M. and Mauer, R. (1974) The anatomy, physiology and biochemistry of the rabbit. In: *The Biology of the Laboratory Rabbit* (eds, Weisbroth, S.H., Flatt, R.E. and Kraus, A.L.), Academic Press, London, pp. 50–69.

Okerman, L. (1994) Inherited conditions and congenital deformities. In: *Diseases of Domestic Rabbits*, 2nd edn, Blackwell Publishing, Oxford, pp. 109–112.

Rush, J.E. and Wingfield, W.E. (1992) Recognition and frequency of dysrhythmias during cardiopulmonary arrest. *Journal of the American Veterinary Medical Association* 200:1932–1937.

# Rabbit Clinics and Owner Education

## 11.1 Rabbit clinics in practice

Rabbit clinics may be something that your practice holds already or may be a completely new concept for you. Rabbit clinics are an ideal means of providing information for owners and prospective owners and hopefully preventing some problems before they start.

Rabbit clinics can run as individual appointments where the rabbit owner can meet with the veterinary nurse. Topics that may be covered include questions about vaccination, worming, grooming, identi-chipping, housing, handling, nutrition, neutering, nail clipping, behaviour, flystrike and preventative treatment. The rabbit can also have its weight monitored on a regular basis. Problems with the rabbit may be identified and the rabbit referred to the veterinary surgeon.

Alternatively, rabbit clinics can involve group appointments where rabbit owners can meet each other. Presentations on specific topics can be given and discussions can take place. This is useful for prospective owners to attend to find out more about what is involved in keeping a rabbit – either outdoors or as a house rabbit.

Special events can be organised by the practice, for example, to tie in with National Rabbit Week or National VN Week. Specific events for children can also be organised. All of these events not only mean that owners are more informed, but also raise the profile of the practice as a rabbit-friendly practice.

## 11.2 Specific topics discussed at a rabbit clinic

We will now look in more detail at some of the more common topics that are discussed at rabbit clinics. It may be useful to prepare handouts for owners to take home with them following their appointment. Examples of care sheets are given in section 11.3. The following, although repeating some of the information already given elsewhere in this book, gives you an idea of some of the commonly asked questions by owners, and short suitable answers to them that may be used in compiling your own information handouts.

### 11.2.1 Husbandry

*What type of housing should rabbits be kept in?*

Housing for your rabbit depends on whether the rabbit will be kept in the house or outside. Rabbits kept outside are usually kept in wooden hutches, which need to be large enough to enable the rabbit to easily turn around and run from end to end. Roughly a minimum hutch size should be 3 times the length of the rabbit by at least 1–2 times the length of the rabbit, unless a run is provided with daily free access. There should be an enclosed bed area and an open run area. The hutch should be raised off the ground and positioned somewhere that is sheltered from rain and wind, but is also not in bright sunshine.

*Can rabbits be kept in the house?*

Yes, rabbits are now commonly kept as house pets. They need to have a bed and toilet area away from children or other animals. They will also chew anything that is at rabbit height, such as wires and potentially poisonous house plants, so these need to be made rabbit proof or hidden from access.

*Should a rabbit be kept on its own, housed with other rabbits,*
*or kept with my guinea pig?*

It is preferable to keep rabbits in pairs or groups rather than singly. They are social animals and benefit from the company of other animals. Pairs of females or neutered males or a neutered male and female work best.

Entire males will often fight as will entire females kept together. However, rabbits can transmit a bacteria (*Bordetella bronchiseptica*) to guinea pigs and rabbits often bully guinea pigs (particularly if the rabbit is an entire male), and therefore it is better not to keep rabbits and guinea pigs together – although there are some owners who have done this without any problems.

## 11.2.2 Nutrition

*What should I feed my rabbit?*

It is important that rabbits receive a high-fibre diet – the simplest way to do this is to provide them with access to fresh hay, dried grass or fresh grass. These grass-based foods should make up the main part of the diet. A pelleted, grass-based food which is homogenous and balanced for calcium and vitamin D3 should also be available. Pellets are better than mixed concentrate because the rabbit will be unable to select sweeter/higher fat parts of the mix and leave other parts as, like humans, rabbits are selective feeders.

*How much should I feed my rabbit?*

Hay, dried grass or fresh grass should always be available. The amount of concentrate to feed your rabbit will depend on the breed of rabbit. Guidelines should be available from the manufacturer. The best thing is to monitor the weight of your rabbit – if an adult rabbit continues to put on weight then too much concentrate is being made available. Fresh, clean water should always be available.

## 11.2.3 Vaccination

*Why does my rabbit need to be vaccinated?*

Two infectious diseases – myxomatosis and viral haemorrhagic disease (VHD) – can now be prevented by vaccination. Both diseases are present in the wild rabbit population in the UK, and have been responsible for the deaths of many pet rabbits. Therefore, it is important to discuss with your practice the likelihood of your pet being affected in the area that you live. As these conditions are fatal in the majority of cases, vaccination is the only form of treatment available.

*How old should my rabbit be when it receives its*
*first vaccinations?*

The age at which rabbits can be vaccinated against VHD depends on
the specific preparation that is being used, and your veterinary practice
can advise. The youngest age at which VHD vaccination can be given
ranges from 5 to 10 weeks (2.5 months) of age.

Rabbits should be at least 6 weeks old before being vaccinated against
myxomatosis.

Vaccination for myxomatosis and VHD cannot be given at the same
time – there needs to be a gap of at least 2 weeks between vaccinations.

*How often do they need to be vaccinated?*

Vaccination for myxomatosis needs to be carried out once or twice a
year, depending on the prevalence of the disease in the area where you
live and whether your rabbit is an indoor or outdoor living one. Your
veterinary practice will be able to advise about this.

Vaccination for VHD is carried out once a year.

## 11.2.4 Worming

*I have heard of worming my dog, but not my rabbit. Why is this?*

Routine worming of rabbits has now become a standard treatment due
to availability of licensed medication.

*What parasites am I worming them for?*

Treatment with an anthelmintic such as fenbendazole will treat rabbits
for nematode worms that are found in the gastrointestinal tract and the
protozoa *Encephalitozoon cuniculi* that can cause kidney and neurological
problems.

*Why is this important?*

*E. cuniculi* infection is regularly identified in rabbits and can be responsible for a variety of clinical signs including nervous system signs, such

as weakness and head tilt, eye problems and kidney disease, and can be fatal. Intestinal nenatode worms may cause diarrhoea particularly in young rabbits.

## 11.2.5 Fleas

*I have heard of flea treatments for my dog and cat but not my rabbit. Why is this?*

Routine flea control in rabbits has become possible due to the availability of safe rabbit-specific medications in the UK.

*What forms of treatment are available for treating fleas in rabbits?*

Currently, there are topical preparations available in the 'spot-on' formulations where a capsule of the drug is emptied onto the skin at the nape of the rabbit's neck. There are different commercial versions available specifically designed for rabbits including preparations containing the adulticide imadacloprid, permethrin-based products and ivermectin-based products which are also designed for dealing with other ectoparasites such as *Cheyletiella parasitivorax*.

*Why is flea treating of my rabbit important?*

Fleas in general are an emotive issue to owners but besides this the rabbit flea (*Spilopysllus cuniculi*) in particular is the vector for myxomatosis. Rabbits are also prone to other fleas, including the dog and cat fleas, and these could also potentially act as vectors for myxomatosis.

## 11.2.6 Common diseases

*What diseases can my rabbit be affected by?*

One of the most common diseases seen in general practice is stasis of the gastrointestinal tract. This is where the rabbit's gut slows down and does not move food along as it should. This can develop if there is an interruption to the usual eating habits of the rabbit. This can be due to food not being available, the rabbit being in pain or any other disease that results in debilitation such as dental disease. Dental disease is more likely in certain breeds, such as the mini lops, dwarf Netherland and others that have a shortened head length, and in rabbits fed a low-fibre, low-calcium/vitamin D3 diet, particularly during their early growing years. Other possible problems are sore hocks (found in rabbits kept on a rough surface, or if they are overweight or are suffering from arthritis), obesity, skin disease, respiratory infections (e.g. *Pasteurella* spp. infection – the cause of rabbit 'snuffles') and abscesses.

### *Why is gastrointestinal disease important?*

Gut stasis can be life-threatening due to a build-up of toxins in the gut from bacteria present there all the time in low numbers. Occasionally, the gut stops working because of a blockage from something the rabbit has eaten, and this too is very serious as rabbits cannot vomit as dogs and cats can, so the blockage is unlikely to be shifted by the rabbit on its own. Therefore, if you see that the rabbit has not eaten anything (or very little) or there is a noticeable reduction in the number of droppings the rabbit is producing during the day or it appears bloated and uncomfortable then you should contact your veterinary practice. Once gut stasis develops it can be a challenging condition to cure.

## 11.2.7 Dental disease

### *What are the signs of dental disease in the rabbit?*

If the problem is with the incisors then it may be possible to see overgrown teeth protruding from the mouth. Problems with the cheek teeth may be more difficult to identify in the early stages. Alternatively, the rabbit may not be eating, the number of droppings it produces may be reduced and there may be sticky pellets accumulating around its rear end. Sometimes, some rabbits will also pull excessive amounts of their fur out when they are suffering from dental pain.

Sometimes though problems with the cheek teeth are only identified by the vet examining the rabbit's mouth, particularly in the early stages.

### *What can be done to treat dental disease?*

The treatment carried out depends on the specific problems that are present. Rabbits' teeth grow continuously and should wear each other down. If there is a problem with the positioning of the teeth so that normal wear does not take place, then it may be necessary to burr back the overgrown teeth using a dental drill. However, as the teeth will continue to grow, this procedure may need to be carried out every few weeks. It is possible in some cases to remove the incisor teeth if these are causing persistent problems.

### *Is there anything I can do to prevent dental disease in my rabbit?*

Some cases of dental disease may be related to the breed or genetics of the individual rabbit – mini lops and dwarf Netherland breeds, for example, are more represented, and it is thought this is due to their shorter head lengths, which inevitably affect the way the teeth wear down against each other. However, it has also been shown that diet plays a large part in the development of dental disease. Making sure that the main part of the rabbit's diet is made up of hay, dried grass or fresh grass is the easiest way of reducing the likelihood of dental disease as well as ensuring, particularly during the growing phase, that rabbits are on a diet with the correct levels of calcium and vitamin D3. However, it is still possible that a rabbit fed such diets could still develop dental disease due to its genetic make-up and of course any traumatic injuries or infections it may encounter throughout its life.

## 11.2.8 Flystrike

### *What is flystrike?*

Flystrike (otherwise known as myiasis) occurs when flies (chiefly the 'bottle' flies) lay their eggs in a wound or in faecally/urine-soaked matted material on the skin of an animal. When the eggs hatch, the larvae eventually will burrow into the flesh of the animal and feed there.

### *How can my rabbit be affected?*

Rabbits are most likely to be affected around the anus due to faecal material and urine gathering there and providing an ideal environment where flies can lay their eggs. Faecal and urine matting is most likely to occur in rabbits that have dental disease, spinal disease or are producing soft faeces due to being fed the wrong diet. A healthy rabbit will rarely develop this problem.

### What can I do to prevent it?

Regularly checking that the rabbit's bottom is clean is the best method of preventing flystrike. If faeces are starting to gather there then they should be removed. If they are not removed easily, then it is best to take the rabbit to the vet, as the skin around this area is very thin and pulling or cutting the faecal material off can result in injury to the rabbit.

Preparations such as Rearguard™ (Novartis) can also be used throughout the summer alongside good husbandry measures. This contains a chemical (cyromazine) that prevents the larvae from developing into the stage which burrows into the flesh. You will therefore still see 'maggots' on the rabbit, but these should not be able to cause the rabbit any damage.

Also, providing the rabbit with a good diet, ensuring that the hutch is kept clean and observing the rabbit for any health problems will reduce the likelihood of your rabbit developing this condition.

## 11.3 Some examples of owner information sheets

The following pages give some examples of the type of information sheets that can be given to owners who have attended a rabbit clinic or who have collected their rabbit after surgery.

# Vaccination of Rabbits

## Background information

Rabbits are routinely vaccinated against two conditions: myxomatosis and VHD. Both of these conditions are present in the wild rabbit population and can be transmitted to your pet. They can cause serious illness and often kill affected rabbits. Therefore, it is important to make sure that your rabbit is vaccinated and that this is kept up to date.

## What is myxomatosis?

Myxomatosis is a viral condition that is spread between rabbits via the rabbit flea. Fleas can spread the condition from wild rabbits or other pet rabbits. Your rabbit does not have to meet other rabbits in order to become infected. Myxomatosis causes swelling of the head and genital area, nose and eye discharges, anorexia (not eating) and depression. Most cases are fatal in unvaccinated rabbits.

## What is VHD?

VHD affects rabbits that are older than 6 weeks of age. It is transmitted by contact between rabbits, or can be carried on clothing, food, bedding or other items that have been in contact with an infected animal. Rabbits can be found dead without previously showing any clinical signs or may show clinical signs such as not eating, depression, laboured breathing, fitting and bleeding from the nose.

## What happens when my pet is vaccinated?

As rabbits are vaccinated against two conditions, they need to be seen on two separate occasions because both vaccines cannot be administered at the same time. Each time the rabbit will be given a small injection under the skin of the scruff. Most rabbits do not notice this. For one of the injections (myxomatosis) some of the vaccine also needs to be given into the skin (intradermally) as well as under the skin.

## How old should my rabbit be when first vaccinated?

Ages vary for the different conditions. The practice policy is:
first vaccination against myxomatosis at _____
first vaccination against VHD at _____

**Does my rabbit need to be vaccinated again?**

Yes, booster vaccinations need to be given to rabbits. Boosters for VHD are given once a year. Boosters for myxomatosis can be given every 6 months or every year. The practice policy is _____

# Neutering of Rabbits

**Background information**

Rabbits become sexually mature (capable of breeding) from 4 to 5 months in the case of males (the buck) and from 5 to 6 months of age in the case of females (the doe). Rabbits are what as known as seasonal breeders. This means that they start to become sexually active at certain times of the year. In the case of most rabbits this is from February/March through to September/October.

**Why should I get my pet rabbit neutered?**

*Males* – In the case of male rabbits, neutering (or castration as it is often called) is important more for behavioural reasons. Entire (non-castrated) males once they become sexually mature can start to mark out their territory, which can include spraying urine. In addition, of course, castration stops successful mating if keeping a buck with an entire doe.

*Females* – In the case of female rabbits, neutering (or spaying as it is often called) is important for many health reasons. The main one is that female rabbits that have not been neutered have a very high incidence (over 80% chance) of womb cancer, which is usually fatal. In addition, neutering helps prevent womb infections (known as pyometras), mastitis (infections of the mammary glands), phantom pregnancies (where the female rabbit develops milk and nest builds but is not actually pregnant) and of course true pregnancy.

In addition, in both sexes, neutering stops the seasonal changes in behaviour, which can involve increased aggression towards other rabbits and owners. Entire males and entire females can fight with their own sex and produce serious injuries during the breeding season, even if they have been kept together since very young ages.

**What age should I get my pet rabbit neutered?**

*Males* – from 4 months of age

*Females* – from 5 months of age

**What is involved in neutering my rabbit?**

*Males* – A full general anaesthetic is required. A castration operation is performed. That means that both testicles are removed, although the scrotum or sac that they sit in is left behind.

*Females* – A full general anaesthetic is required. An ovariohysterectomy is performed. This means that the uterus (womb) and the ovaries are removed in an operation that requires making a small wound in the belly of the doe.

Usually the stitches used in both operations are implanted beneath the skin surface and so cannot be seen after the operation. These dissolve of their own accord over the next few weeks after the surgery.

# Insurance for Rabbits

### Background information

There is unfortunately no national health service for animals. However, it is possible for a relatively small amount of money to insure many pets against the day they require veterinary treatment. It is now possible to insure rabbits as well as other domestic pets.

### Why should I insure my rabbit?

There are many more things that fortunately can be done to help your pet rabbit should he/she become ill. With advancing technology and techniques, inevitably there has been some increase in cost and it is a relief to know that decisions regarding your rabbit's health can be made without concerns regarding costs of the procedures.

### What things can I insure my rabbit for?

It is possible to insure your rabbit against most eventualities and the level of this cover as with all insurance policies depends on the type of policy you initially take out. Universally, however, there are some things that insurance policies do not cover and these can include the following:

- Vaccination
- Routine flea treatment and worming treatment
- Routine neutering (castration and spaying)
- Normal diets such as adult or growing rabbit pelleted foods

It is best to refer to the policy document for the insurance company you choose and discuss your requirements with your prospective insurer and your veterinary practice.

### Who provides insurance for rabbits?

There are a number of insurance companies that now cater for insuring rabbits. Your veterinary practice can give you leaflets and further information regarding the range of policies available.

# Flea Treatment and Worming of Rabbits

**Background information**

Rabbits, like cats and dogs, can suffer from fleas and other ectoparasites (external or skin parasites such as mites) as well as worms and other endoparasites (internal parasites). Some of these are rarely a problem, but they can build up in numbers to cause a potential problem, and some can cause serious disease or transmit serious disease to the rabbit.

**Why should I treat my pet rabbit for fleas and other ectoparasites?**

Rabbits can suffer from the rabbit flea (*Spillopsyllus cuniculi*) which attaches around the ear tips, and other fleas which can affect cats and dogs. The rabbit flea in particular is a concern for rabbits kept outside for part or all of the year as these are transmitted from wild rabbits and can carry the virus myxomatosis which can be fatal in unvaccinated rabbits.

**What products are available?**

There are a range of products available in the UK to treat fleas and other ectoparasites in rabbits. They are often in a so-called spot-on form as you may be familiar with for dogs and cats. This is where the contents of a small capsule are applied to the skin on the nape of the neck. The compound then spreads over the whole of the body, killing fleas wherever they are on the rabbit. IT IS VITALLY IMPORTANT THAT THE RABBIT VERSION OF THE PRODUCT IS USED AND NOT CAT OR DOG ONES. This is to avoid overdosage which can be fatal with some of the chemicals used. The chemicals that are used are often based on permethrins or use other parasiticides such as ivermectin or imidacloprid. Many of these compounds are also effective against other ectoparasites such as the dandruff mite *C. parasitivorax* and so may be prescribed by your vet for other reasons than fleas.

**Why should I treat my pet rabbit for worms and other endoparasites?**

Some rabbits that have regular access to outside runs may pick up gastrointestinal worms. These may not cause problems in small numbers, but they can build up to large levels in some individuals, particularly the young and the older rabbits, and cause loss of body condition and recurrent gut problems.

There is another endoparasite that can cause severe problems – the microscopic *Encephalitozoon cuniculi*, often shortened to *E. cuniculi* for obvious reasons. This parasite can cause neurological and kidney disease and is transmitted from rabbit to rabbit by close contact or from mother to the kitten at the time of birth.

### What products are available?

There are specific rabbit-formulated wormers available on the market in the UK, based on the drug fenbendazole. This particular drug also helps to treat *E. cuniculi*, although the dosage used and frequency of dosage are different. Your veterinary surgeon will be able to discuss this with you further if he/she has diagnosed *E. cuniculi* infection.

# Dietary Requirements for Rabbits

### Background information

Rabbits are strict herbivores. That means they only eat vegetable matter and in reality the 'wild-type' diet of the European rabbit from which all domestic rabbits are descended is largely based on grass with a few leafy greens and the occasional root vegetable at certain times of the year thrown in. This needs to be borne in mind when feeding your pet rabbit as obesity, dental disease and gut upsets are all likely sequels to an inappropriate diet.

### What is the dietary requirement for my growing rabbit?

As mentioned above, it is important to ensure that the predominant portion of the diet is based on grass. This of course may be presented as dried grass or good quality meadow hay for the indoor/house rabbit. Growing rabbits also require an increased level of calcium and vitamin D3 in comparison with adult ones to allow proper bone growth and avoid some dental problems later in life. For this reason there are commercial pelleted diets available that are designed for growing rabbits, although they should be fed with hay/dried grass/fresh grass rather than instead of it.

### What is the dietary requirement for my adult pet rabbit?

Adult rabbits should be fed a high-fibre diet largely based around good quality hay, dried grass or fresh grazed grass. It is important if feeding fresh grass that this is not cut and then fed to rabbits, as this can result in fermentation within the rabbit's gut and subsequent bloating. Instead, the rabbit should be allowed to graze the grass directly. This high-fibre diet is essential to allow: stimulation of the gut; wearing of the teeth which are continuously growing and can overgrow without adequate abrasion; and to provide a source of nutrition for the normal micro-organisms present in the rabbit's gut to provide food for the rabbit and prevent abnormal potentially dangerous micro-organisms from being able to grow. Such a diet may be supplemented with a commercial dry food for rabbits in small amounts. It is preferable when feeding such a dry food that a pelleted homogenous diet is fed to prevent the rabbit from selectively eating only one portion of the diet. Alternatively, if feeding a loose mixed diet, only enough of it should be given in a day so that the rabbit eats all of it without leaving any part of the mix. This is the only way to ensure that not only is a balanced diet offered to the rabbit but that the rabbit actually eats a balanced diet.

**What treats are safe to give to my pet rabbit?**

It is advisable to avoid all sugary, high-fat and high-protein treats. Therefore, human sweet biscuits, dog and cat foods, and of course any animal meat or dairy products should be avoided. Chocolate should also be avoided as it is harmful to rabbits.

Foods that may be fed as treats include small amounts of root vegetables such as carrot; fresh dandelion leaves; small amounts of high-fibre human savoury biscuits and commercially prepared treats specifically designed for rabbits.

# Postoperative Recovery Sheet for Rabbits

**Operation details**

Your rabbit has just undergone a general/local* anaesthetic and an operation.

The operation performed was _____

The operation was performed by _____ MRCVS/FRCVS*

The anaesthetic was monitored by _____ RVN MBVNA*

**What should I be looking for in my pet rabbit?**

Your rabbit may be slightly lethargic after his/her* operation. It is important to keep an eye on the wound for any signs of bleeding, swelling or for any evidence that the wound is opening up.

It is also important that your rabbit is watched closely for the first 24 hours to ensure that he/she* is eating, drinking, and passing droppings and urine as normal. A slight reduction in all of the above is to be expected, but serious reductions should be immediately reported to the veterinary practice.

**What should I feed my pet rabbit after his/her operation?**

It is important to offer the usual foods your rabbit is used to after surgery as familiarity will help a quicker return to appetite.

**What medications should I be giving to my pet rabbit?**

Your rabbit has undergone an anaesthetic and surgery as detailed above. As a result of this he/she* will need/not need* ongoing medication:

**Details of ongoing medication:**

Please give the following medication _____ as directed on the label.

This drug has been dispensed for the following reason _____

**When should I bring my pet rabbit back for a check-up?**

Your rabbit should be brought back to the veterinary practice for a check-up with the veterinary surgeon/veterinary nurse* to check his/her* progress in _____ days. Please make an appointment with our receptionist or with the veterinary surgeon/veterinary nurse on discharge.

*Delete as appropriate.*

# Research and Evidence-Based Medicine

## 12.1 Implementation of evidence-based medicine in practice

*Evidence-based medicine* is a term which you will hear mentioned more and more in the veterinary nursing press, but what exactly does it mean?

Think for a moment about how you know what to do with a rabbit that comes into the practice. Did you learn this at college or university? Did another member of staff within the practice tell you what to do? Did you learn this from a textbook such as this one? But have you ever thought about where the information came from in the first place?

Evidence-based medicine is a method by which the procedures that we carry out in practice have been shown through research studies to be the best. This does not necessarily mean that they will be any different to the way in which something has 'always been done', but we have the knowledge that they have been shown to be the best method.

In order to keep up with the changes in evidence-based medicine, you need to keep up with your reading and professional development. Reading research and review papers and attending lectures will keep you up to date with recent advances, but the heart of evidence-based medicine is that any article or lecturer will be able to support their claims with the original research.

However, research alone is not the Holy Grail. We hope that all or at least most research papers out there are founded on scientific principles and that the claims they are making are seen to be true. Unfortunately, there may be times when this is not the case. Therefore, you need to be able to make a judgement on a research paper and decide for yourself if you believe the claims that they are making. There are a number of factors which help you in this, which we now examine.

## 12.2 Theory of research

### 12.2.1 Qualitative and quantitative research

Before you can assess a research paper, it is helpful to know something about how research is carried out and reported. In its broadest terms, research can be divided into two main groups: qualitative and quantitative. Qualitative research describes those studies which are interested in the feelings and emotions of its subjects. Qualitative research reports trends and usually contains quotes from the subjects. Therefore, a qualitative study can be carried out on owners' animals as we can ask them how they feel, but we cannot carry out a qualitative study on animals as obviously we cannot ask them their opinion.

Quantitative research uses numbers to report the findings, either measuring something, for example, a laboratory test, or describes the results of a questionnaire in a numerical form. For example, a research paper may describe that 55% of respondents gave a particular answer – this would be a quantitative piece of work.

Quantitative research can be further described according to the type of study, from descriptive to experimental as detailed in Table 12.1. Terminology used within research can appear confusing. Some explanations of the more commonly used terminology are given in Table 12.2.

### 12.2.2 Sampling

*Sampling method*

Any research needs a population to study – whether this is people, animals or bacteria. The way in which the sample is selected will have a dramatic effect on the results. If we want to be able to apply our results to the population as a whole, then the sample needs to be representative of that population. There is no point in carrying out a research project where we only look at Netherland dwarf rabbits and then try to apply our results to every other breed of rabbits.

Possible sample selection methods are as follows:

1. Include all available data
2. Random sampling
3. Convenience sampling

**Table 12.1** Types of quantitative research

| Description | Definition | Advantages | Disadvantages |
|---|---|---|---|
| Descriptive | As the name suggests, this research describes a particular topic. For example, the frequency with which rabbits are anaesthetised with isoflurane in general practice | Accurate<br>Can provide new information about a topic | Does not provide any information about the relationship between different factors |
| Correlational | This type of research looks for a link between two or more factors. For example, the association between nutrition and the development of dental disease in rabbits | Examines the relationship between factors | Does not determine cause and effect |
| Quasi-experimental | Examines cause and effect, but variables are not controlled. An example of this type of study could be a clinical trial in practice, where rabbits undergoing surgery were given an analgesic preoperatively. If all rabbits undergoing surgery were included in the study rather than restricting the study to a particular age then this would quasi-experimental | Can provide more information than a descriptive study | Does not involve as much control as an experimental study. Therefore, results are less powerful |
| Experimental | Examines cause and effect. Any variables within the study are controlled in the design of the study. For example, the provision of analgesia to laboratory rabbits where the age, species and type of procedure are all controlled by the researcher | Can examine cause and effect. Variables are controlled, so results are most powerful. Can enable the researcher to predict outcomes | Difficult and costly to run |

**Table 12.2** Definitions of terminology used in research

| Description | Definition | Advantages | Disadvantages |
|---|---|---|---|
| Retrospective study | Examines historical data | Data has already been collected so studies can be carried out in a shorter time | As the data has already been collected, there is may be no control over how the information is gathered |
| Prospective study | Examines data collected during a study | The study is designed and then data collected accordingly so there is control over the type of data collected | There is no room for change in the study or the gathering of extra information |
| Random sample | A method of ensuring that every member of the population has an equal chance of being included in the research | Results are representative of the population | May be costly and time-consuming |
| Convenience sample | Sample is selected due to its availability to the researcher | Low cost. Useful where there is limited time for a study | Results may not be representative of the population as a whole |

1. **Include all available data**

   Where a population is small then it may be possible to include all available data. For example, if you wanted to find out the rate of postoperative complications in rabbits neutered in your practice, then you could include all of the patients treated in the past 2, 5 or 10 years. However, the results could only then be applied to your practice. They could not be applied to any other practice. However, they may enable you to identify areas of good (hopefully not bad) practice, which could be adopted by other practices.

2. **Random sampling**

   The basis of random sampling is that every member of the population has an equal chance of being included in the research. To ensure that the sample is random, chance needs to be used when allocating participants. So picking names out of hat or selecting names at random form a list can be used. This is a bit like a lottery.

3. **Convenience sampling**

   Convenience sampling is not a random process and therefore is not a representative of the population. Convenience sampling relies on the availability of participants. Samples such as these may be used where there is limited time or limited funds to carry out a study.

*Size of sample*

The size of the sample is also important. The larger the sample size, the more likely it is that the results are due to a true effect rather than chance. However, how big should a sample be? This is a very difficult question to answer and involves the use of statistics, which is beyond the scope of this book. In human studies it is not unusual to see studies that include hundreds or thousands of people. It is very difficult within veterinary medicine to carry out studies on this scale, and therefore most veterinary studies are much smaller than human equivalents. It is though still important for the studies to be as large as possible. Any examination of veterinary literature will reveal the tendency for case reports to be published where a small number of cases or even one case is described. Whilst the information and results contained within these papers can be perfectly valid, they should be read with caution – just because a particular finding was reported in one animal does not mean that it will be the case for the general population.

*Sample population characteristics*

For anyone in practice, the research needs to be able to be applied to animals in the general population. Therefore, it is preferable that the sample comes from a similar population. Information gained from a particular breed in a laboratory may well be applicable to all breeds of rabbits, but it is possible that it may not.

When reading a study, the sample and sampling method should be described. Questions to ask here include the following:

- Where did the sample come from?
- Is the sample the same as the population I deal with?
- What is the age range of the sample (narrow or broad)?
- Are all the subjects male, female or equally distributed?
- Were all subjects healthy?
- If not, did all subjects suffer from the same problem?
- Were any other problems present in some but not all subjects?

If you feel that the researcher has answered all of these questions, and you can see that the conclusions from their research can indeed be applied to the general population, then you can feel confident in their results. If, however, the answers to these questions mean that the data cannot be applied to the general population, you may have to take care in applying these results to general practice.

### 12.2.3 Ethics

Any published research paper should identify the ethical implications of the work, and whether ethical approval was granted and by whom. However, in many veterinary papers this is not mentioned as it is assumed that ethical approval would have been given and therefore does not need to be mentioned. Further information on ethics is given Section 12.4.

## 12.3 Questions to ask when reading a research paper

1. **What type of research has been carried out?**
   Is this a quantitative study or a case report?
2. **What sampling method was used?**
   Was the sample random?
   How did they ensure that it was random and not biased?
3. **How large was the sample studied?**
   Was the sample in single figures, tens, hundreds or thousands?
4. **Was the sample representative of the population?**
   Are the characteristics of the sample similar to those of the general population?
5. **What results were obtained?**
   Are the results clear? Can you identify the results?
6. **Did the conclusions agree with the results?**
   It is not unusual for clinicians (veterinary nurses and veterinary surgeons) to be pushed for time. If you ever get time to read a research paper, then it will usually involve reading just the abstract, or reading the introduction and the conclusion. However, if you find that this work is something that is of interest to you, might be something that you can do in practice, or relates to a case that you are dealing with at the moment, then it is worthwhile going back through the paper and just making sure that you agree with the conclusions arrived at by the researcher. It is important to make sure that you are

happy with the findings before you decide to implement the findings in your own work.

7. **Were there any flaws in the research, or anything about the design that you would change?**
   Is there anything about the research that, had you been carrying out the project, you would have done differently?

8. **How appropriate is this research for implementation in practice?**
   Is the research applicable to practice? If the research has been carried out in a laboratory then it is possible that it may be useful in practice.

## 12.4 Do you want to carry out your own research?

Before carrying out some form of research, the ethical aspects of the research need to be examined. If your research is part of a project for a university then that institution will have an ethics committee, which will have to review your proposal before you are allowed to carry out the work. If you intend to carry out research within the practice, such as reviewing the number of cases of dental disease in rabbits, which the practice has seen over the last year, then you have to justify the ethics to yourself. Any research comes under the remit of the following:

The Guide to Professional Conduct for Veterinary Nurses 2007
The Data Protection Act 1998
The Animals (Scientific Procedures) Act 1986

Therefore, you are not allowed to carry out a procedure on a patient which would not normally be carried out as part of their treatment. So, for example, if you were interested in the packed cell volume of rabbits receiving fluid therapy, you would not be allowed to take a blood sample from that animal specifically for research purposes as this would come under the remit of experimentation and you would need a Home Office licence. However, you could examine historical records from patients who have passed through the practice. Confidentiality, however, needs to be maintained, and the permission of the senior partner of the practice would need to be obtained before records could be examined. If the research is part of clinical audit and therefore just for the use of the practice, for example, reviewing the incidence of postoperative infections following rabbit spays, then it would not be necessary to obtain owner permission. However, if you wished to publish this research then it would be advisable to obtain permission to include patients within the study. It is essential that all results are anonymous and that your records are stored safely.

It is possible to carry out research by way of questionnaire – for example, to find out more about owner knowledge or owner opinions. Again the permission of the practice principal would be required before embarking on this. When undertaking an owner questionnaire, it is necessary to complete an information sheet detailing the aims of the research and a consent form which the participant must sign. You need to recognise that owners may change their mind and they must be allowed to withdraw from the research if they so wish. Again anonymity is necessary, so names should not be attached to any questionnaires.

## 12.5 Areas of future research

The most successful areas of research are those which are of interest to the researcher. There is no point in deciding to carry out research into the underlying causes of sore hocks in your rabbit patients if you are more interested in the clinical presentations of dental disease. Thinking about the common conditions that you see in your practice will give you some ideas about areas that could be researched further. Also questioning why you do something may well lead to some clinical research. If you do not know why you do something then chances are that many other veterinary nurses are in the same situation.

Research within veterinary nursing, rather than veterinary medicine, is still in its infancy and there are many aspects of nursing care which we give to our patients, which are copied from human nursing, often without any theoretical grounding.

Why not have a think about this during your next coffee break?

## Further reading

Burns, N. and Grove, S. (2003) *Understanding Nursing Research*, 3rd edn, Saunders, Pennsylvania.

Cockcroft, P. and Holmes, M. (2003) *Handbook of Evidence Based Veterinary Medicine*, Blackwell Publishing, Oxford.

Petrie, A. and Watson, P. (1999) *Statistics for Veterinary and Animal Science*. Blackwell Publishing, Oxford.

The Royal College of Nursing, Research & Development Co-ordinating Centre – http://www. man.ac.uk/rcn/

# Appendix 1: Formulary

NB: In the following tables the symbols have the following meanings: SC, subcutaneous; PO, per os; IV, intravenously; IO, intra-osseously; IM, intramuscularly; IP, intraperitoneally; q, every (e.g. q6 hours means 'once every 6 hours')

**Table 1** Antimicrobial drugs

| Antimicrobial | Dosage | Notes |
|---|---|---|
| Ciprofloxacin | 5–20 mg/kg PO q12 hours | Particularly effective against *Pasteurella* spp. |
| Clotrimazole | Use topically | Useful against ringworm. Do not use with cisapride |
| Doxycycline | 2.5 mg/kg PO q12 hours | |
| Enilconazole | Topically every third day | Dilute to 1:50 solution with water |
| Enrofloxacin | 5–10 mg/kg PO, SC q12 hours | Licensed in the UK for rabbits as Baytril® (Bayer) |
| Fusidic acid | Topically as eyedrops 1–2 drops q12–24 hours | Licensed in the UK for rabbits as Fucithalmic® (Leo) |
| Gentamicin | Topically as eyedrops 1–2 drops q8–12 hours | Licensed in the UK for rabbits as Tiacil® (Merial) |
| Griseofulvin | 25 mg/kg PO q24 hours for 14–45 days | Treatment of ringworm. Do not use in pregnant does as teratogenic |
| Metronidazole | 20–30 mg/kg PO q12 hours | Treatment of choice for enterotoxaemia |
| Oxytetracycline | 15 mg/kg SC, IM q24 hours 100–125 mg/L drinking water | Useful for treating *Clostridium piliforme* (Tyzzer's disease) |
| Oxytetracycline (long-acting depot injection) | 30 mg/kg SC once | |
| Penicillin G | 40 000 IU/kg SC once, repeat after 5–7 days on one or two occasions | Treatment of rabbit syphilis. May be used q24 hours with care for some sensitive bacterial infections |
| Trimethoprim-sulphonamide | 30 mg/kg PO q12 hours 30 mg/kg SC q24 hours | Not licensed for use in rabbits in the UK but a human palatable oral syrup is available, making administration easier |

**Table 2** Antiparasitic drugs

| Antiparasitic | Dosage | Notes |
|---|---|---|
| Albendazole | 15–20 mg/kg PO q24 hours for 2–3 weeks | Treatment of *Encephalitozoon cuniculi*. Potentially teratogenic |
| Cyromazine | Apply topically as 6% solution every 8–10 weeks | Prevents conversion of L1–L2 larvae of blow flies |
| Fenbendazole | 20 mg/kg PO q24 hours for minimum 3 weeks (*E. cuniculi*)<br>10–20 mg/kg PO once, repeat in 2 weeks (for nematodes) | Treatment of choice for *E. cuniculi* |
| Imidacloprid | 10 mg/kg topically | Licensed for use in preventing fleas in the UK |
| Ivermectin | 0.2–0.4 mg/kg PO, SC every 10–14 days on three occasions<br>1:10 dilution with propylene glycol and spray onto affected site for maggots (keep overall dose ivermectin below 0.4 mg/kg) | Most ectoparasites, particularly mites<br>Also spot-on preparations now licensed for use in the UK |
| Permethrin | Topical treatments | Preparations now licensed for use in the UK for flea and lice treatment |
| Praziquantel | 5–10 mg/kg PO, SC, IM repeat in 10 days | Injections may cause muscle necrosis. Used as anti-cestode |
| Selamectin | 6–18 mg/kg topically once | Useful for mites but not licensed |
| Toltrazuril | 25 mg/kg PO q24 hours for 2 days, then repeat after 5 days<br>Or<br>25 mg/L drinking water for 5–7 days | Coccidiosis particularly for *Eimeria stiediae* which may be resistant to other anti-coccidials |
| Trimethoprim-sulphonamide | 40 mg/kg PO q12 hours | Coccidiosis |

**Table 3** Anaesthetics and analgesics

| Anaesthetics and analgesics | Dosage | Notes |
|---|---|---|
| Acepromazine | 0.1–0.5 mg/kg SC | Premedication |
| Buprenorphine | 0.01–0.05 mg/kg SC, IV, IM q6–12 hours | Analgesic |
| Butorphanol | 0.1–0.5 mg/kg SC, IM, IV q2–4 hours | Analgesic |
| Carprofen | 2–4 mg/kg PO, SC q24 hours | Analgesic and anti-inflammatory |
| Hypnorm® (fentanyl/ fluanisone) | 0.1–0.5 mL/kg | Provides light to moderate sedation. Useful as premed to prevent breath-holding during gaseous induction. Licensed for use in rabbits in the UK. Reversal of Hypnorm with butorphanol or buprenorphine to speed recovery |
| Hypnorm + diazepam | 0.3 mL/kg Hypnorm + 2 mg/kg diazepam IP or IV | Separate syringes as the two drugs do not mix. Provides surgical anaesthesia. Reversal of Hypnorm with butorphanol or buprenorphine to speed recovery |
| Hypnorm + midazolam | 0.3 mL/kg Hypnorm + 2 mg/kg midazolam IP or IM | Reversal of Hypnorm with butorphanol or buprenorphine to speed recovery |
| Isoflurane | Gradual stepwise induction with 100% oxygen. Usually 1.5–2% isoflurane for maintenance (see Chapter 6) | Licensed for use in rabbits in the UK |
| Ketamine + medetomidine | 15 mg/kg ketamine + 0.25 mg/kg medetomidine SC | Short procedure anaesthesia |
| Ketamine + medetomidine + butorphanol | 5 mg/kg ketamine + 0.05 mg/kg medetomidine + 0.5 mg/kg butorphanol IV Or 10 mg/kg ketamine + 0.2 mg/kg medetomidine + 0.5 mg/kg butorphanol SC (takes 10–15 minutes to work) | Provides surgical anaesthesia for short procedures. May be reversed with atipamezole at 1 mg/kg. Advisable with all these combinations to intubate and provide oxygen |
| Meloxicam | 0.2–0.6 mg/kg PO, SC q24 hours | Analgesic and anti-inflammatory |
| Morphine | 2–5 mg/kg SC, IM q2–4 hours | Can cause moderate-to-severe respiratory depression |
| Sevoflurane | Can induce at 4% sevoflurane in 100% oxygen. Maintenance at 2–3% sevoflurane (see Chapter 6) | Better tolerated as gaseous induction agent than isoflurane |

**Table 4**  Miscellaneous drugs

| Drug | Dosage | Notes |
|---|---|---|
| Calcium EDTA | 27.5 mg/kg SC q6 hours for 5 days | Treatment of lead poisoning. Fluid therapy essential |
| Cholestyramine | 2 g/20 mL drinking water for 14–21 days Or 500 mg/kg orally q12 hours | Treatment of enterotoxaemia as binds toxins in the gut and prevents absorption |
| Cisapride | 0.5–1 mg/kg PO q12–24 hours | Becoming more difficult to source in the UK |
| Dorzolamide hydrochloride | Topically 1–2 drops q8–24 hours | Eyedrops for treating glaucoma |
| Furosemide | 5–10 mg/kg IM q12 hours | Lower dosages can be given IV (1–4 mg/kg) |
| Glycopyrrolate | 0.02 mg/kg SC, IM | Use for profound bradycardia and in preference to atropine due to serum atropinesterases in 60% of rabbits |
| Metoclopramide | 0.2–0.5 mg/kg PO, SC q4–8 hours | Can be used with ranitidine to promote intestinal motility |
| Nandrolone | 0.5–2 mg/kg | Anabolic steroid as supportive therapy for chronic renal failure and hepatic lipidosis |
| Oxytocin | 0.1–3 IU/kg SC, IM | Encourage uterine contractions when birth canal is not obstructed but delayed parturition has occurred. Also aids milk let-down |
| Povidone-iodine | Dilute 1:25 with water | Can be used as general antiseptic or for nail bed fungal infections |
| Prednisolone | 0.25–0.5 mg/kg PO q12 hours for 3 days, then q24 hours for 3 days and finally q48 hours | Rabbits are very sensitive to the side effects of corticosteroids and these should be avoided where possible |
| Proligestone | 30 mg/kg PO q 24–48 hours | For pseudopregnancy to stop milk production |
| Ranitidine | 2–5 mg/kg PO q12 hours | Prokinetic and antacid. Use with metoclopramide as synergistic |
| Silver sulfadiazine | Apply topically q12–24 hours | Effective against *Pseudomonas aeruginosa* (blue fur disease) amongst other infections |
| Vitamin A | 500–1000 IU/kg PO, IM once | Oral administration potentially safer |
| Vitamin B complex | 0.02–0.4 mL/kg IM q24 hours | |
| Vitamin B1 | 1–2 mg/kg IM | Thiamine deficiency or where neurological disease exists |
| Vitamin B12 | 20–50 $\mu$g/kg IM | Chronic renal failure as appetite stimulant |
| Vitamin C | 50–100 mg/kg PO | May inhibit toxin production and can aid caecotrophy |
| Vitamin E/selenium | 12.5 mg (17 IU)/rabbit IM | |
| Vitamin K | 1–10 mg/kg PO, SC | |

EDTA, ethylene diamine tetra acetic acid.

# Appendix 2: Some Common Garden and House Plants Poisonous to Rabbits

| Plant | Toxin | Clinical signs/pathology |
|---|---|---|
| Aconite (aka monkshood) | Alkaloid (aconitine) | Gastrointestinal (GI) irritant, small amounts can be fatal |
| Anemones | Anemonin | GI irritant and can cause blisters in the mouth. May result in paralysis if eaten in large enough quantities |
| Arum family | Unknown poison | Berries, leaves and possibly flowers poisonous |
| Box | Alkaloid (buxine) | GI irritant |
| Buttercups and other members of the Ranunculus family (e.g. kingcups and celandines) | Protoanemonin | Irritant to the GI tract |
| Cabbage (if fed in large quantities) | Goitrogens | Induce goitre |
| Clematitis | Protoanemonin | GI irritant and diuretic |
| Daffodils and other amaryllis plants | Alkaloids | Unlikely poisoning as leaves bitter, but consumption of bulbs can also be poisonous, producing purgative effects |
| Cyclamen | Glycoside (cyclamin) | Salivation, increased heart rate and respiration with diarrhoea |
| Deadly nightshade, woody nightshade and henbane | Atropine and allied alkaloids | Not all rabbits susceptible due to presence of atropinesterases in 60%. Can cause tachycardia and mydriasis |
| Delphinium | Alkaloids | GI irritant, erratic heart rate |
| Dieffenbachia | Oxalates | GI irritant skin erythema |
| Foxglove | Cardiac glycoside (digitalis) | Cardiac arrhythmias |
| Hellebore | Alkaloids | Bloody diarrhoea and excessive urination. Erratic heart rate |
| Hemlock | Alkaloid (conine) | Paralysis, reduced respiration and heart rate. No convulsions |

*(continued)*

| Plant | Toxin | Clinical signs/pathology |
| --- | --- | --- |
| Ivy | Unknown | GI irritant. Unlikely to be eaten in large enough quantities to be poisonous |
| Laburnum | Alkaloids | Seeds more toxic, collapse and anorexia |
| Lily of the valley | Alkaloids | GI irritation, cardiac arrhythmias |
| Lupin | Alkaloids and quinolizidine | Garden varieties generally low toxicity but may cause GI irritation and cardiac arrhythmias |
| Mistletoe | Glycoside | GI irritant, diarrhoea, rapid heart rate and respiration |
| Poinsettia | Saponin alkaloids | Oral and GI irritant with salivation and diarrhoea |
| Privet | Heteroside Tannins | GI irritant, lethal in small quantities |
| Rhododendrons, laurels and azaleas | Andromedotoxin | Rabbits may be resistant to the poison except in large quantities |
| St John's wort | Flavenoids | Photosensitisation, potentially depressive effects in large quantities |
| Woody nightshade | Atropine | Not all rabbits susceptible due to presence of atropinesterases in 60%. Can cause tachycardia and mydriasis |
| Yew | Taxine (an alkaloid) | Cardiac toxin |

# Appendix 3: Useful Organisations

British Veterinary Zoological Society
Caters for vets and vet nurses interested in rabbits, exotic pets, and zoo
    and wildlife
Contact:
Mr D. Lyon
7 Bridgwater Mews
Gresford Heath
Pandy
Wrexham LL12 8EQ
http://www.bvzs.org

Rabbit Welfare Association & Fund
PO Box 603
Horsham
West Sussex
RH13 5WL
http://www.houserabbit.co.uk

Burgess Supafeeds
PO Box 38
Pickering
YO18 7YH

Fur and Feather
Elder House
Chattisham
Ipswich
Suffolk
IP8 3QE
http://www.furandfeather.co.uk

# Index

Printed and bound by CPI Group (UK) Ltd, Croydon, CR0 4YY